# Sudden Cardiac Death

Editor

Alessandro Capucci MD
Division of Cardiology
Guglielmo da Saliceto Hospital
Piacenza
Italy

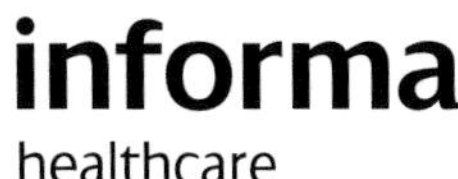

First published in the United Kingdom in 2007 by Informa Healthcare, 4 Park Square, Milton Park, Abingdon, Oxon OX14 4RN. Informa Healthcare is a trading division of Informa UK Ltd. Registered Office: 37/41 Mortimer Street, London W1T 3JH. Registered in England and Wales number 1072954.

Tel: +44 (0)20 7017 6000
Fax: +44 (0)20 7017 6699
Email: info.medicine@tandf.co.uk
Website: www.informahealthcare.co.uk



A CIP record for this book is available from the British Library.

Library of Congress Cataloging-in-Publication Data

Data available on application

ISBN-10: 1 84184 578 7
ISBN-13: 978 1 84184 578 4

Distributed in North and South America by
Taylor & Francis
6000 Broken Sound Parkway, NW, (Suite 300)
Boca Raton, FL 33487, USA

*Within Continental USA*
Tel: 1 (800) 272 7737; Fax: 1 (800) 374 3401
*Outside Continental USA*
Tel: (561) 994 0555; Fax: (561) 361 6018
Email: orders@crcpress.com

Distributed in the rest of the world by
Thomson Publishing Services
Cheriton House
North Way
Andover, Hampshire SP10 5BE, UK
Tel: +44 (0)1264 332424
Email: tps.tandfsalesorder@thomson.com

Composition by C&M Digitals (P) Ltd, Chennai, India
Printed and bound in Great Britain by Antony Rowe Ltd, Chippenham, Wiltshire

Dedicated to my son and daughter, Gianluca and Sara and to my young old friend Elisabetta.

# Contents

# Contributors

**Daniela Aschieri** MD
Division of Cardiology
Guglielmo da Saliceto Hospital
Piacenza
Italy

**Gust H Bardy** MD
Clinical Professor of Medicine
Attending Physician
University of Washington Medical Center
Seattle, WA
USA

**Matteo Bertini** MD
Institute of Cardiology
University of Bologna
Bologna
Italy

**Mauro Biffi** MD
Institute of Cardiology
University of Bologna
Bologna
Italy

**Giuseppe Boriani** MD PhD
Institute of Cardiology
University of Bologna
Bologna
Italy

**Angelo Branzi** MD
Institute of Cardiology
University of Bologna
Bologna
Italy

**Günter Breithardt** MD PhD FESC FACC FHRS
Professor of Medicine (Cardiology)
Head of Department of Cardiology and Angiology
Hospital of the University of Muenster
Münster
Germany

**Alessandro Capucci** MD
Division of Cardiology
Guglielmo da Saliceto Hospital
Piacenza
Italy

**Nicola Carano** MD
Department of Pediatrics, Pediatric Cardiology
University of Parma
Parma
Italy

**Erga L Cerchiari** MD
Department of Anesthesia and Intensive Care
Hospital Maggiore
Bologna
Italy

**Paolo Della Bella** MD
Arrhythmia Department
Institute of Cardiology
University of Milan
Cardiological Center Monzino
IRCCS
Milan
Italy

**Igor Diemberger** MD
Institute of Cardiology
University of Bologna
Bologna
Italy

**Giulia Domenichini** MD
Institute of Cardiology
University of Bologna
Bologna
Italy

**Lars Eckardt** MD PhD
Department of Cardiology and Angiology
Hospital of the University of Muenster
Münster
Germany

**Cecilia Fantoni** MD
Department of Cardiovascular Sciences
Circolo e Fondazione Macchi Hospital
University of Insubria-Varese
Varese
Italy

**Raffaella Marazzi** MD
Department of Cardiovascular Sciences
Circolo e Fondazione Macchi Hospital
University of Insubria-Varese
Varese
Italy

**Cristian Martignani** MD PhD
Institute of Cardiology
University of Bologna
Bologna
Italy

**Carlo Napolitano** MD PhD
Senior Scientist, Molecular Cardiology
IRCCS Foundation Salvatore Maugeri
Pavia
Italy

**Jeanne E Poole** MD
Associate Professor of Medicine/Cardiology
University of Washington School of Medicine
Division of Cardiology
Seattle, WA
USA

**Silvia G Priori** MD PhD
Molecular Cardiology Laboratories
IRCCS Foundation S Maugeri
Pavia
Italy

**Claudio Rapezzi** MD
Institute of Cardiology
University of Bologna
Bologna
Italy

**Benjamin J Rhee** MD
Spokane Cardiology, PSC
Spokane, WA
USA

**Stefania Riva** MD
Arrhythmia Department
Institute of Cardiology
University of Milan
Cardiological Center Monzino
IRCCS
Milan
Italy

**Jorge A Salerno-Uriarte** MD
Department of Cardiovascular Sciences
Circolo e Fondazione Macchi Hospital
University of Insubria-Varese
Varese
Italy

**Federico Semeraro** MD
Department of Anesthesia and Intensive Care
Maggiore Hospital
Bologna
Italy

**Umberto Squarcia** MD
Department of Pediatrics, Pediatric Cardiology
University of Parma
Parma
Italy

**Cinzia Valzania** MD
Institute of Cardiology
University of Bologna
Bologna
Italy

**Kristina Wasmer** MD
Department of Cardiology and Angiology
Hospital of the University of Mueuster
Münster
Germany

**Matteo Ziacchi** MD
Institute of Cardiology
University of Bologna
Bologna
Italy

# Preface

Sudden cardiac death (SCD) accounts for about 50% of all cardiovascular mortality in developed countries with a survival rate of 1–2% despite modern health service provision. Early defibrillation with very simple automatic or semiautomatic machines is nowadays feasible and affordable by almost everyone, and could enhance survival to more than 10–20%. Today, however, there is a lack of interest from the medical and scientific community in this issue. While the mass media, politicians, and the scientific community are appalled by cancer and rare diseases, SCD is not considered as shocking despite being the "silent killer" of the Western world.

During my professional life, I have observed too many patients die suddenly and too many relatives asking me why this event happened. I was personally shocked by the loss of a lovely friend who died at 29 years of age. Since the time for intervention must be very short (no more than 5 minutes), all the actors in the survival chain need to have a few but sharp ideas on how to act. The community has to be involved as the first link of the chain, and therefore has to know the signs of imminent SCD. Moreover, they need to know how important it is to immediately call an ambulance for first aid and to waste no time finding the nearest external defibrillator.

In this book, my aim has been to summarize our present understanding of SCD in a comprehensive way and to give some practical information on the care and management of one particular group of patients: those who will potentially die suddenly. This book is intended for medical students, house officers, practicing physicians, and emergency providers who treat patients at risk of SCD both inside and outside hospital. Many friends and expert physicians wrote all the chapters in a simple and comprehensive way and I thank them all.

Ample space has been devoted to the definition of SCD, its epidemiology, and the size of the problem, as well as the correct clinical and instrumental identification of patients at risk. Primary prevention is also a mainstay in the treatment of patients at risk, and this has been extensively treated, with a review of the main clinical trials.

International experiences have been reported on the issue of first aid, advanced life support, and post-resuscitation care, according to recent guidelines. Early defibrillation must be considered the standard of care for potential adult victims of SCD. Pediatric SCD and its genetic basis has also been treated by experts in the field.

A particular effort has been made to provide an up-to-date bibliography, and the book includes more than 500 references, and a substantial number of tables and figures to support the text.

I hope not only that you will find this book a guide to your clinical practice but also that it will enable those in medical practice to remember to make the defibrillation process a quick and extended procedure in all communities.

I acknowledge with gratitude the authors who have contributed with their insight, time, and talents to this educational initiative. Our goal is to help save the lives of relatives and friends of all of you.

AC

# Introduction

Alessandro Capucci

Sudden cardiac death (SCD) is a consequence of abrupt loss of heart function (i.e. cardiac arrest) in a person who may or may not have previously diagnosed heart disease; time and mode of death are unexpected, and it occurs instantly or shortly after the onset of symptoms.[1] SCD is mainly the end result of untreated rapid ventricular tachycardia or ventricular fibrillation,[2] or of extreme slowing of the heart.[1] While previous heart disease is a recognized risk factor for SCD, an individual may have no history or symptoms of heart disease prior to the onset of SCD.

Despite recent progress in the management of cardiovascular disorders and in particular of cardiac arrhythmia, sudden cardiac death remains both a problem for the practicing clinician and a major public health issue.[1–3] Estimates of the number of SCDs that occur in the USA each year range from 250 000 to 500 000;[1,3] 125 000 deaths annually in the USA alone occur in people with no history of heart disease. SCD usually occurs without early warning, away from hospitals. In Europe, the rate of about one SCD per 1000 inhabitants has also been confirmed in recent trials.[4] Death comes quickly, usually within minutes or hours.

Despite advances in the prevention and treatment of heart disease and improvements in emergency transport, the rate of SCD remains high, probably because of its unexpected nature and the failure to recognize early warning symptoms and signs of heart disease. The age-adjusted SCD rates and the state-specific variation in the percentage of SCD suggest a need for increased public awareness of heart attack symptoms and signs. Early recognition of heart symptoms and signs leads to earlier artery opening treatment or defibrillation that results in less heart damage and deaths. Education and media efforts should inform the public about heart disease symptoms and signs; this is particularly important for women and young adults, who might dismiss heart disease as a problem of men and the elderly.[5] Healthcare providers should be alert for atypical symptoms of heart disease among female and young adult patients.

Reduction in mortality from SCD involves two issues: prevention and treatment of underlying risk factors, and interruption of SCD events through rapid defibrillation of the heart and eventually basic life support (BLS) or advanced cardiac life support (ACLS) maneuvers. Several early defibrillation projects in the community have been set up in the last decade, with positive results in the percentage of saved lives and a clear reduction of SCD due to ventricular fibrillation. The rate of saved patients improved from 1–2% in controls to 4–5% in the actual early defibrillation project. The number is positive, but far from arousing enthusiasm. We think therefore that new ideas and consequently new directions are needed in the fight against this hidden and powerful enemy.

The underlying causes of SCD are varied, and sometimes unknown. Some of the known causes include cardiac ischemia, abnormal electrical conduction in the heart, structural abnormalities of the heart, atherosclerosis of the coronary arteries, and changes in the heart due to long-standing hypertension. The risk factors generally accepted as being associated with heart disease include family history of heart disease, increased age, being male, hypertension, increased blood cholesterol, cigarette smoking, and diabetes. The main three risk factors that increase the risk of SCD are history of previous myocardial infarction, depressed left ventricular ejection fraction, and presence of complex ventricular ectopy.

Many recent trials have pointed out the great importance of early recognition and time to intervention in order to save lives. But what kind of intervention is appropriate, and how can time be saved? It is still a matter of debate whether early defibrillation is the most effective initial intervention or whether it should be secondary to basic life support maneuvers, although the most recent guidelines from the European Resuscitation Council[5] lean toward the later approach. In addition, the interest of the mass media and of politicians and decision-makers in the issue of SCD has been somewhat sporadic in recent years, with attention generally being confined to specific high-profile cases. This is unfortunate, given the prevalence of SCD and the potential importance of public access defibrillation (PAD) programs. Although the number of such programs has increased in recent years, a lack of specific medical support, poor planning, and insufficient collection of data have had a negative effect and have lessened the political impact of these programs.

Another important issue arises from the fact that more than 80% of SCDs occur at home – therefore, if we want to save some 50% of these lives by defibrillating within 5 minutes, it is essential that there be widespread and easy access to automatic external defibrillator (AED) equipment. One possibility, applicable at least within urban areas, is for each large building (e.g. an apartment block) to have an easily accessible fully automated AED that could be used by any person, even without specific training.

It is the aim of this book to consider and tackle the many questions related to the topic of SCD – some of them contentious – in the hope that their solution will be of great help in saving more lives in the future.

## REFERENCES

1. Epstein FH, Pisa Z. International comparisons in ischemic heart disease mortality. Proceedings of the Conference on the Decline in Coronary Heart Disease Mortality. NIH Publication No. 79-1610. Washington, DC: US Government Printing Office, 1979: 58–88.
2. Gillum RF. Sudden coronary death in the United States: 1980–1985. Circulation 1989; 79: 756–65.
3. Report of the Working Group on Arteriosclerosis of the National Heart, Lung, and Blood Institute. Vol 2: Patient Oriented Research – Fundamental and Applied, Sudden Cardiac Death. NIH Publication No. 83-2035. Washington, DC: US Government Printing Office, 1981: 114–22.
4. Capucci A, Aschieri D, Piepoli MF, et al. Tripling survival from sudden cardiac arrest via early defibrillation without traditional education in cardiopulmonary resuscitation. Circulation 2002; 106: 1065–70.
5. Handley AJ, Koster R, Monsieurs K, et al. European Resuscitation Council Guidelines for Resuscitation 2005: Section 2. Adult basic life support and use of automated external defibrillators. Resuscitation 2005; 67(Suppl 1): S7–23.

# 1

# What is sudden death? A correct identification

Jorge A Salerno-Uriarte, Cecilia Fantoni
and Raffaella Marazzi

## DEFINITION: TRULY SUDDEN DEATH OR AFTER A RELATIVELY SHORT TIME FROM THE ONSET OF HEART DISEASE

'Sudden cardiac death is a natural death due to cardiac causes, heralded by abrupt loss of consciousness within one hour of the onset of acute symptoms; preexisting heart disease may or may not have been known to be present, but the time and mode of death are unexpected.'[1] This is the apparently easy and clear definition of sudden cardiac death (SCD), almost universally accepted and used in the most recent guidelines. It contains and underlines all the following important elements that are necessary to define a death as 'sudden cardiac death':

- *Natural event*: it is a biological event, so that all the violent and accidental causes have to be excluded.
- *Cardiac*: even if, rarely, the primary cause of this event could lie elsewhere than in the heart, the final cause of such an event is always an abrupt cessation of cardiac pump function with consequent abrupt loss of cerebral blood flow.
- *Rapid*: the time elapsed between the onset of symptoms signaling the abnormalities directly responsible for the cardiac arrest and the cardiac arrest itself should be less than 60 min. The window time frame previously used to describe the duration of the final event was 24 h, but it has been reduced to 1 h or even to an instantaneous event (within 5 min from onset of acute symptoms) in order to render an arrhythmic mechanism more likely. Nevertheless, although it is true that most cases of instantaneous deaths are arrhythmic in origin, there are many other mechanisms that can lead to death within a few minutes. On the other hand, not all the life-threatening arrhythmic events result in death or cause instantaneous death.
- *Unexpected*: the death appears in a person without any prior condition that would appear fatal in the short time.

In spite of this apparently easy and clear description, there is still an important matter of debate on the best definition regarding the following key points:

- How can a death be defined as primarily cardiac? In reality, everybody dies finally due to cardiac arrhythmia (asystole or ventricular fibrillation) even if the primary condition leading to death is noncardiac. How can we know the remote and primary cause of a death without necroscopy or sophisticated postmortem studies? Many times, the real background leading to a fatal arrhythmia is unknown, so that a sudden death is defined erroneously as cardiac. Almost all cases of unexpected and rapid-evolving natural death are defined as SCD, without any effort to define the primarily cardiac nature of such events.

- Since most of the cases of SCD occur out of hospital and in the absence of witnesses, how can we define the real timing of such an event? How can we know when the patient was last alive and for how long he suffered from symptoms that led to his sudden death? For example, almost all cases of people found dead in bed are arbitrarily defined as SCD, even if the timing of these fatal events is completely unknown and could not fit the real definition of SCD.
- Are most cardiac deaths really unexpected? Since most of the cases of SCD occur in patients with an underlying heart disease that carries a high risk of arrhythmia, can we call the sudden fatal events really unexpected? Nevertheless, in more than 30% of patients dying suddenly, SCD constitutes the first symptom of heart disease, and the death is unexpected because of our ignorance or failure to recognize the underlying disease.

## SUDDEN DEATH AND ADJUSTABLE CAUSES

Adjustable causes of SCD refer to all those conditions that can be responsible for SCD and that, once recognized and corrected, permit avoidance of the fatal event. Big efforts have been directed in the last decades to identify all the theoretically adjustable causes of SCD in order to prevent it.

The single most important cause of SCD among adults is coronary artery disease, with or without previous myocardial infarction, accounting for more than 75% of cases of SCD.[2] Nevertheless, different pathophysiologic mechanisms involved in coronary artery disease can cause SCD. The most important distinction is that between acute and chronic ischemic phenomena that can lead to SCD. All together the causes of SCD related to coronary artery disease can be avoided by preventing or at least limiting coronary artery disease in its severity; that is, by controlling the risk factors.

Once ischemic heart disease has begun, many processes directly responsible for SCD can be prevented or at least treated in order to reduce maximally the risk of sudden fatal events. Silent or symptomatic myocardial ischemia has to be promptly recognized and corrected in order to avoid the onset of acute coronary syndrome, while all the acute ischemic events have to be rapidly and effectively treated in order to limit to the maximal extent the degree of irreversible myocardial injury. Since it has been demonstrated that, after an acute ischemic event has stabilized, post-infarction scars, together with ventricular enlargement and depression of left ventricular function, constitutes the most important substrate for the onset of ventricular tachyarrhythmia due to a re-entry mechanism, efforts have to be made to slow disease progression, such as to limit the reverse remodeling process after a myocardial infarction. Prompt correction of residual myocardial ischemia and pharmacologic treatment seem to be the best available means to do this. Finally, in the chronic post-infarction phase of ischemic heart disease, the elimination of an arrhythmogenic substrate via a surgical approach (aneurysmectomy) or trans-catheter ablation can completely resolve the issue.

Among other adjustable causes of SCD, myocarditis seems to account for around 5% of out-of-hospital SCD, mainly among young people.[3] Two patterns have to be distinguished: the acute form, involving mainly children or young adults, is characterized by patchy inflammatory infiltrates and injured myocardial cells exhibiting easily triggered activity, and the chronic form, mainly characterized by patchy areas of fibrosis with consequent slow-conduction phenomena, resulting in arrhythmogenic substrate for re-entry circuits. Prompt recognition and treatment of acute myocarditis limit both the acute and chronic arrhythmogenic phenomena.

In patients with Wolff–Parkinson–White syndrome, SCD occurs due to degeneration into ventricular fibrillation of a fast-conducted atrial fibrillation through the atrioventricular accessory pathway. Among these patients, the annual SCD rate has been estimated to be about 0.15%. Patients at highest risk of SCD are those presenting with short R-R intervals during atrial fibrillation and multiple accessory pathways. An electrophysiologic evaluation of the R-R interval during induced atrial fibrillation seems to have high sensitivity, but poor specificity and positive predictive value in identifying patients at highest risk.[4] Transcatheter ablation of the accessory pathway completely abolishes the risk of sudden death in these patients.

Severe aortic stenosis accounts for a very small number of cases of SCD, mainly in old people. Among all patients dying of aortic stenosis, death is sudden in about 20% of cases. Unfortunately, no instrumental or clinical parameter has been demonstrated to be useful in identifying patients with aortic stenosis at highest risk of fatal arrhythmia. Valve replacement, always recommended in symptomatic patients, completely abolishes the risk. The anomalous origin of the left main coronary artery from the right or the noncoronary sinus of Valsalva accounts for a small number of cases of SCD among young patients, so that particular attention should be turned to young patients complaining of angina. Also in these patients, surgical intervention completely resolves the issue.[5]

Many electrolyte imbalances, such as hypo- or hyperkalemia, that can pathologically affect the depolarization and repolarization processes may also lead to life-threatening ventricular arrhythmia in an otherwise healthy heart. Such a risk is particularly relevant in patients with an underlying structural cardiac disease or treated with drugs that can affect by themselves the electrolyte balance. Furthermore, many agents, such as many antiarrhythmic drugs, can have a proarrhythmic effect, mainly by prolonging the QT interval and inducing 'torsade de pointes'.

## SUDDEN DEATH AND UNADJUSTABLE CAUSES

Unadjustable causes of SCD refer to all those conditions that are responsible for SCD and that, even if recognized, cannot be corrected. In these cases, prevention of SCD lies in the prompt recognition and interruption of life-threatening arrhythmia, mostly through the implantation of a cardioverter defibrillator.

SCD is the single most common cause of death in patients with nonischemic dilated cardiomyopathy. Given the relatively high number of patients affected by dilated cardiomyopathy, the identification of patients at highest risk of fatal arrhythmia is mandatory. Few parameters have been recognized as good predictors of SCD, but left ventricular ejection fraction ($\leq$40%) has been demonstrated to be the most accurate one,[6] while occurrence of syncopal events is the second most accurate one,[7] followed by ventricular conduction disturbances (QRS duration at the ECG $\geq$120 ms). The risk of SCD related to systolic dysfunction is not linear, but shows a big increase when the left ventricular ejection fraction falls below 40%. The risk of SCD related to functional NYHA class gains relative importance in classes I–II, compared to classes

III–IV, where death from heart failure is predominant. Even if pharmacologic treatment with ACE inhibitors, beta-blockers, aldosterone antagonists and amiodarone has significantly reduced mortality from any cause and also mortality due to SCD of patients with nonischemic dilated cardiomyopathy, the risk of SCD remains high, particularly among patients with left ventricular ejection fraction below 30%.[8]

Hypertrophic cardiomyopathy, with an estimated prevalence of 1:500, constitutes a relatively common cause of SCD among young asymptomatic patients.[9] Major attention must be directed to the early diagnosis of this severe heart disease and to the correct identification of the small subset of patients with hypertrophic cardiomyopathy that are at high risk of SCD. A correlation seems to exist between the degree of ventricular wall hypertrophy and the incidence of SCD. It has been estimated that a wall thickness of 30 mm or more is associated with a cumulative 20-year risk of SCD of about 40%.[10] Other important prognostic factors include a family history of cardiac arrest or recurrent syncope. The apical variant of hypertrophic cardiomiopathy seems to be associated with a minimal risk of SCD.[11]

Arrhythmogenic right ventricular cardiomyopathy is another important cause of SCD in the precoronary artery disease age group. Although predictive markers of SCD have not yet been clearly identified in large prospective studies, SCD seems to occur more frequently in patients with extensive right ventricular changes and in those with left ventricular involvement.[12]

Congenital long QT syndrome in all its variable phenotypes is a rare syndrome associated with high risk of developing SCD. Risk stratification is mainly based on genetic characterization and history of syncope or cardiac arrest,[13] while the duration of the corrected QT interval is not a good predictor of SCD in these patients. Genetic defects of the sodium channel gene (LQT3) usually carry a higher risk of SCD than defects of the potassium channel gene (LQT1 and LQT2).

Brugada syndrome is another rare cardiac disorder responsible for unexpected, fatal arrhythmic events, mainly in middle-age men. Since up to 80% of the victims had previously experienced a syncope, high-risk patients have to be considered all the patients with a typical Brugada ECG and a history of syncope.[14]

Short QT syndrome[15] is a rare, recently identified, arrhythmogenic disorder, associated with a mutation of the genes encoding for different potassium channels. Patients affected by short QT syndrome present with a variable clinical pattern, ranging from mild symptoms, such as palpitations, to syncope and SCD. SCD may occur at any age, sometimes even in children in the first months of life and very often it constitutes the first symptom of this disorder. A value of 340 ms for the QTc interval has been proposed as the cut-off for the diagnosis of short QT syndrome.

Among other rare, arrhythmogenic, inherited disorders, catecholaminergic polymorphic ventricular tachycardia (CPVT)[16] has recently gained growing interest. CPVT occurs in a structurally normal heart, mostly as a bidirectional VT, or more rarely as a polymorphic VT, both easily and reproducibly inducible during exercise or catecholamine infusion. Usually, CPVT is associated with a familiar history of syncope and/or juvenile SCD. According to genetic analysis of affected patients, CPVT seems to be linked to mutations of the genes encoding for an intracellular ion channel, controlling calcium handling.

## SUDDEN DEATH AND TRUE FIRST EVENT

The complexities of SCD range from the absence of a precise and uniform definition over time of what should be classified as SCD to the epidemiologic uncertainty of a definition of the true incidence of SCD. The latter problem is increased by the incompleteness of the registries of sudden deaths. In fact, surveys about incidence rates are based on victims in whom resuscitation was attempted, therefore excluding unwitnessed sudden deaths. Moreover, autopsy, which allows identification of true cases of SCD, is performed in only a small percentage of victims. These uncertainties make it difficult to discuss the problem with evidence-based data. Registries including all cases of SCD, witnessed and unwitnessed, preferably with a postmortem diagnosis of the cause of death, would allow us to obtain better insight into the true incidence of sudden cardiac arrest outside the hospital, the profiles of the victims, the exact causes of death and the effect of interventions to resuscitate the victims.[17]

The most common sequence of events leading to SCD appears to be the degeneration of fast ventricular tachycardia (VT) into ventricular fibrillation (VF), causing disorganized and ineffective contractions of the ventricles, often followed by asystole or pulseless electrical activity. In fact, the first recorded rhythm in patients with a sudden cardiovascular collapse is VF in 75–80% of cases. Bradyarrhythmia and electromechanical dissociation (EMD) contribute as first event to the remaining cases of SCD.[18] The occurrence of severe tachyarrhythmia, bradyarrhythmia or asystole is the end of a cascade of pathophysiologic abnormalities which result from complex interactions between coronary vascular events, myocardial injury, variations in autonomic tone, and/or the metabolic and electrolyte state.[1]

The magnitude of the risk of fatal arrhythmia is both age- and disease-related. The risk of SCD, at 1–2 per 1000 inhabitants per year,[19] shows the most marked increase at the age of 40–65 years, according to the high prevalence of coronary artery disease (CAD) in that subgroup of the population accounting for about 75% of all SCDs. Cardiomyopathy is responsible for 10–15%. Among patients with advanced, frequently unknown, structural heart disease, the extent of the disease rather than the age determines the risk; therefore, age-related risk curves tend to blunt in that subgroup of the population. Adolescents and young adults (aged 10–30 years) have a risk of SCD of about 1 per 100 000 individuals annually (about 1/100 that of the general adult population), with a modest inverse age relationship, giving the adolescent group a higher mortality risk than young adults. It is likely that the risk of fatal arrhythmia in the genetically controlled disorders, such as hypertrophic cardiomyopathy, long QT syndrome, arrhythmogenic ventricular cardiomiopathy and Brugada syndrome, tends to appear more commonly in the adolescent years.[1]

Acquired functional and structural changes occurring in the diseased, whether silent or known, heart as well as genetic factors (e.g., mutations of ion-channel-encoding genes, polymorphism of beta-adrenergic receptors) may contribute to an increased risk of dying suddenly. The nature of the immediate precipitating event that triggers the fatal ventricular tachyarrhythmia at a specific time in an otherwise stable patient remains the major point of interest. The concept of response variables is an attempt to introduce principles of epidemiology to the discipline of cardiac electrophysiology. It refers to the mechanism by which a specific individual who has a structural basis of risk, such as CAD or cardiomyopathy, is susceptible to arrhythmogenesis when exposed to a transient functional influence. The epidemiologic question focuses on the identification of those subjects whose characteristics make the initiation of electrophysiologic instability more likely when these conditions are met. Individual risk predictors, such as acquired or genetically based features, might provide even greater resolution for SCD risk stratification in specific individuals.[1] Recent studies suggested familial clustering of cardiac arrests as a specific clinical expression of acute coronary events that might derive from genetic predisposition.[20]

A series of possible gene mutations or polymorphisms that do not affect baseline phenotype, but do express effects during a transient event, have been provided.[21] This individual-specific risk might explain why patients with similar risk factors for CAD may suffer from SCD or nonfatal ischemic events.

The importance of recognizing the principle that the very high-risk patient categories represent only a very small part of the universe of SCD risk highlights that the benefits reported by the clinical trials of implantable defibrillators[22–27] apply only to these small studied subgroups, while finding specific risk markers for the magnitude of the population may emerge as having potential to improve public health. To achieve this goal, new approaches for risk stratification will be required.[1]

## LIFE-THREATENING TACHYARRHYTHMIAS

The transient risk factors (ischemia and reperfusion, hemodynamic and metabolic factors, autonomic fluctuations, and pharmacologic and toxic cardiac effects) are the functional transient events that have the potential to trigger and maintain an unstable electrophysiologic condition. Transient pathophysiologic changes can convert ventricular myocardium from a stable to an unstable state (susceptible myocardium) at a specific time, permitting the genesis of fatal arrhythmia and creating a link between acute pathophysiologic changes and chronic abnormalities. In the absence of myocardial vulnerability, many triggering events, such as frequent and complex premature ventricular beats, may be innocuous. Intense functional changes alone may destabilize this system in the absence of structural abnormalities, but the vast majority of cardiac arrests occur in hearts with preceding structural abnormalities.[1]

Since the large majority of SCDs are associated with CAD, the distribution of chronic arterial narrowing has been well defined by previous studies.[28] Steady-state reductions in regional myocardial blood flow, in the absence of superimposed acute lesions, could create a setting in which alterations in the metabolic or electrolyte state of the myocardium, or neural fluctuations, result in loss of electrical stability.[29] Increased myocardial oxygen demand with a fixed supply may be the mechanism of exercise-induced arrhythmia and sudden death during intense physical activity in athletes or others whose heart disease had not previously been clinically manifested.[30] Vasoactive events leading to acute reduction in regional myocardial blood flow in the presence of a normal or previously compromised circulation constitute a common cause of transient ischemia, angina pectoris, arrhythmia, and possible SCD. Coronary artery spasm exposes the myocardium to the double hazard of transient ischemia and reperfusion.[31,32] The mechanism of spasm production is unclear, although sites of endothelial disease appear to be predisposing.[33] A role of the autonomic nervous system, even if it does not seem to be a sine qua non, has been suggested.[34] Vessel susceptibility and humoral factors, particularly those related to platelet activation and aggregation, also appear to be important mechanisms.[35] Transition of stable atherosclerotic plaques to an 'active' state due to endothelial damage, with plaque fissuring leading to platelet activation and aggregation followed by thrombosis, appears to contribute to SCD during acute ischemia. In addition to initiating the thrombus, platelet activation produces a series of biochemical alterations that may enhance or retard susceptibility to VF by means of vasomotor modulation.[36] In a very high percentage of subjects who died suddenly, acute coronary thrombi and/or plaque fissuring were evident, but only 18% of these patients had more than

75% stenosis.[37] Moreover, the discrepancy between the relatively high incidence of acute thrombi in postmortem studies and the low incidence of new myocardial infarction among survivors of out-of-hospital VF highlights this question.[38] Spontaneous thrombolysis, a dominant role of vasospasm induced by platelet products, or a combination of both mechanisms may explain this discrepancy.[1]

At the level of the myocyte, the onset of acute ischemia produces immediate electrical (reduction of transmembrane potentials, enhanced automaticity), mechanical (loss of effective contractile function) and biochemical (efflux of $K^+$, influx of $Ca^{++}$, acidosis) dysfunction. The slow conduction and electrophysiologic instability that occur regionally in the ischemic myocardium, adjacent to nonischemic tissue, create a setting for re-entry, and thus possible re-entrant arrhythmia. Premature impulses generated in this environment may further alter the dispersion of recovery between ischemic tissue, chronically abnormal tissue, and normal cells, leading to complete electrical disorganization and finally VF. VF is not only a consequence of re-entry, since rapidly enhanced automaticity caused by ischemic injury to the specialized conducting tissue or triggered activity in partially depolarized tissue may result in rapid bursts of automatic activity that also could lead to failure of coordinated conduction and onset of VF.[39] Experimental studies also have provided data on the long-term consequences for tissue exposed to chronic stress produced by left ventricular pressure overload[40] or tissue healed after ischemic injury.[41] They both show basic cellular electrophysiologic abnormalities, including regional changes in transmembrane action potentials and refractory periods, so that acute ischemic injury in the presence of healed myocardial infarction is more arrhythmogenic than in previously normal tissue.[42] Reperfusion of ischemic areas due to spontaneous thrombolysis, collateral flow from other vascular beds or reversal of vasospasm may sustain some mechanisms of reperfusion-induced arrhythmogenesis that appear to be related to the duration of ischemia prior to reperfusion.[43,44] The continuous influx of $Ca^{++}$ may determine electrical instability and induce afterdepolarizations as a triggering response for $Ca^{++}$-dependent arrhythmia. Formation of superoxide radicals[45] is also recognized as a possible mechanism of reperfusion arrhythmia, while different endocardial and epicardial muscle activation times and refractory periods[46] may be involved in both ischemia and reperfusion electrical instability.

The association of metabolic and electrolyte abnormalities, as well as neurophysiologic and neurohumoral changes,[47] with SCD increases the myocardial substrate propensity to fatal arrhythmia.

## BRADYARRHYTHMIA AND ASYSTOLE

Bradyarrhythmic and asystolic arrests are more common in severely diseased hearts and probably represent diffuse involvement of subendocardial Purkinje fibers. Anoxia, acidosis, shock, renal failure, trauma and hypothermia, all systemic influences that increase extracellular $K^+$ concentration, may result in partial depolarization of normal or already diseased pacemaker cells, with a decrease in the slope of spontaneous phase 4 depolarization and ultimate loss of automaticity.[48] Functionally depressed automatic cells are more susceptible to overdrive suppression, so that brief bursts of tachycardia may be followed by prolonged asystolic periods, with further depression of automaticity by the consequent acidosis and increased local $K^+$ concentration, or by changes in adrenergic tone. The ultimate consequence may be degeneration into VF or persistent asystole.[1]

EMD, that is pulseless electrical activity, refers to continuous electrical activity of the heart in the absence of effective mechanical function. It can be secondary to acute mechanical obstruction of flow, acute disruption of a major blood vessel, cardiac tamponade, or rupture of the ventricle. In primary EMD, mechanical events are absent, but ventricular muscle fails to produce an effective contraction despite continuous electrical activity (failure of electromechanical coupling).[49] It usually occurs as an end-stage event in advanced heart disease, but it may also occur in patients with acute ischemic events or, more commonly, after electrical resuscitation from prolonged cardiac arrest.

## CLINICAL AND INSTRUMENTAL FEATURES

Studies from Seattle[50] and from Miami[38] demonstrated that only a minority of survivors of out-of-hospital cardiac arrest had evidence of a new transmural myocardial infarction, thus leading to the conclusion that in the majority of such patients, transient pathophysiologic events were responsible for cardiac arrest.

Prodromal symptoms, such as chest pain, dyspnea, weakness or fatigue, palpitations, and a number of unspecific complaints, may presage coronary events, particularly myocardial infarction and SCD. Nonetheless, a minority (31–46% in different studies[51,52]) of victims of SCD consulted the medical system weeks to months before SCD, and only a small subgroup of them (from one-third[51] to one-fourth[52]) had consulted a physician because of symptoms which appeared to be related to the heart. A history of previous infarction and congestive heart failure complicating the infarction is useful to identify patients at increased mortality risk, although this is not specifically predictive of SCD. In these patients, many tests are available and are mandatory to stratify risk of SCD, including those that assess nonarrhythmic parameters, such as the presence of residual myocardial ischemia, functional status (exercise test) and left ventricular function (echocardiograms and gated blood pool scans). Ambulatory ECG monitoring assesses the presence and extent of spontaneous arrhythmia, which is presumed to trigger and initiate VT and/or VF. Tests to detect the presence of a substrate for ventricular tachyarrhythmia include signal-averaged ECG, measurement of QT dispersion, T-wave alternans and invasive electrophysiologic studies. Finally, a third group of tests evaluating abnormalities of the autonomic nervous system, which modulates the interactions between the presumed triggers and the arrhythmogenic substrate, is represented by heart rate variability and baroreflex sensitivity.[53]

Limited information is available about the clinical status at the 'onset of the terminal event' (the period of 1 h before the cardiac arrest). Fortuitous monitor recordings indicate increasing heart rate and advancing grades of ventricular ectopies before VF, but no parallel clinical symptoms are equally documented.[54] The cardiac arrest itself is characterized by abrupt loss of consciousness owing to inadequate cerebral blood flow, due to VF/VT, bradyarrhythmia/asystole or EMD, events which lead to death in the absence of active intervention, since spontaneous reversion is rare. The potential for successful resuscitation is a function of the setting in which cardiac arrest occurs, the mechanism of the arrest, and the clinical status of the victim.

In survivors of cardiac arrest, the clinical features are heavily influenced by the type and extent of the underlying disease associated with the event. An instrumental evaluation of these patients is necessary to define both the adequate therapy and their risk profile. A time-dependence of recurrence among survivors of cardiac arrest has been well described. Among a population of 101 cardiac arrest survivors with CAD, the risk was highest in the first 6 months (11.2%) and then fell to 3.3%/6 months for the next three 6-month blocks. After 24 months, the rate fell to 0.8%/6 months. A low ejection fraction was the most powerful predictor of death during the first 6 months; subsequently, persistent inducibility during programmed stimulation, despite drug therapy or surgery, was the most powerful predictor.[55]

## REFERENCES


1. Myerburg RJ, Castellanos A. Cardiac arrest and sudden death. In: Braunwald E, ed. Heart Disease: A Textbook of Cardiovascular Medicine. 6th edn. Philadelphia: WB Saunders, 2001: 890–931.
2. Holmes DR Jr, Davis KB, Mock MB et al. The effect of medical and surgical treatment on subsequent sudden cardiac death in patients with coronary artery disease: a report from the Coronary Artery Surgery Study. Circulation 1986; 73: 1254–63.
3. Lecomte D, Fornes P, Fouret P et al. Isolated myocardial fibrosis as a cause of sudden cardiac death and its possible relation to myocarditis. J Forensic Sci 1993; 38: 617–21.
4. Zipes DP, Di Marco JP, Gillett PC et al. Guidelines for clinical intracardiac electrophysiological and catheter ablation procedures. A report of the American College of Cardiology/American Heart Association Task Force on Practice Guidelines. J Am Coll Cardiol 1995; 26: 555–73.
5. Click RL, Holmes DR, Vlietstra RE et al. Anomalous coronary arteries location, degree of atherosclerosis and effect on survival – a report from the Coronary Artery Surgery Study. J Am Coll Cardiol 1989; 13: 531–7.
6. Keogh AM, Baron DW, Hickie JB. Prognostic guides in patients with idiopathic or ischemic dilated cardiomyopathy assessed for cardiac transplantation. Am J Cardiol 1990; 65: 903–8.
7. Knight BP, Goyal R, Pelosi F et al. Outcome of patients with nonischemic dilated cardiomyopathy and unexplained syncope treated with an implantable defibrillator. J Am Coll Cardiol 1999; 33: 1964–70.
8. Bardy GH, Lee KL, Mark DB et al for the Sudden Cardiac Death in Heart Failure Trial (SCD-HeFT) Investigators. Amiodarone or an implantable cardioverter-defibrillator for congestive heart failure. N Engl J Med 2005; 352: 2225–37.
9. Maron BJ, Olivoto I, Spirito P et al. Epidemiology of hypertrophic cardiomyopathy-related death: revisited in a large non-referral-based patients population. Circulation 2000; 102: 858–64.
10. Sprito P, Bellone P, Harris KM et al. Magnitude of left ventricular hypertrophy and risk of sudden death in hypertrophic cardiomyopathy. N Engl J Med 2000; 342: 1778–85.
11. Eriksson MJ, Sonnenberg B, Woo A et al. Long-term outcome in patients with apical hypertrophic cardiomiopathy. J Am Coll Cardiol 2002; 39: 638–45.
12. Corrado D, Basso C, Thiene G et al. Spectrum of clinico-pathologic manifestations of arrhythmogenic right ventricular cardiomyopathy/dysplasia: a multicenter study. J Am Coll Cardiol 1997; 30: 1512–20.
13. Zareba W, Moss AJ, Schwartz PJ et al. Influence of genotype on the clinical course of the long-QT syndrome. International Long-QT Syndrome Registry Research Group. N Engl J Med 1998; 339: 960–5.
14. Brugada J, Brugada R, Brugada P. Right bundle-branch block and ST-segment elevation in leads V1 through V3: a marker of sudden death in patients without demonstrable structural heart disease. Circulation 1998; 97: 457–60.
15. Gaita F, Giustetto C, Biauchi F, et al. Short QT syndrome. a familial case of sudden death. Circulation 2003; 108: 965–70.
16. Leenhardt A, Lucet V, Denjoy I, et al. Catecholaminergic polymorphic ventricular trachycardia in children. A seven–year follow up of 21 patients. Circulation 1995; 91: 1512–
17. Wellens HJJ, Gorgels AP, de Munter H. Sudden death in the community. J Cardiovasc Electrophysiol 2003; 14(Suppl): S104–7.

18. Priori SG, Aliot E, Blømstrom-Lundqvist C et al. Task Force on Sudden Cardiac Death, European Society of Cardiology. Summary of recommendations. Europace 2002; 4: 3–18.
19. Becker LB, Smith DW, Rhodes KV. Incidence of cardiac arrest: a neglected factor in evaluating survival rates. Ann Emerg Med 1993; 22: 86–91.
20. Jouven X, Desnos M, Guerot C, Ducimetiere P. Predicting sudden death in the population: the Paris Prospective Study I. Circulation 1999; 99: 1978–83.
21. Kubota T, Shimizu W, Kamakura S, Horie M. Hypokalemia-induced long QT syndrome with an underlying novel missense mutation in S4–S5 linker of KCNQ1. J Cardiovasc Electrophysiol 2000; 11: 1048–54.
22. Moss AJ, Hall WJ, Cannom DS et al. The Multicenter Automatic Defibrillator Implantation Trial Investigators: improved survival with an implanted defibrillator in patients with coronary disease at high risk for ventricular arrhythmia. N Engl J Med 1996; 335: 1933–40.
23. The Antiarrhythmic versus Implantable Defibrillators (AVID) Investigators: a comparison of antiarrhythmic-drug therapy with implantable defibrillators in patients resuscitated from near-fatal ventricular arrhythmias. N Engl J Med 1997; 337: 1576–83.
24. Connolly SJ, Gent M, Roberts RS et al. The CIDS Investigators: Canadian Implantable Defibrillator Study (CIDS): a randomized trial of the implantable cardioverter defibrillator against amiodarone. Circulation 2000; 101: 1297–1302.
25. Buxton AE, Lee KL, Fisher JD et al. A randomized study of the prevention of sudden death in patients with coronary artery disease. Multicenter Unsustained Tachycardia Trial Investigators. N Engl J Med 1999; 341: 1882–90.
26. Kuck KH, Cappato R, Siebels J, Ruppel R. Randomized comparison of antiarrhythmic drug therapy with implantable defibrillators in patients resuscitated from cardiac arrest: the Cardiac Arrest Study Hamburg (CASH). Circulation 2000; 102: 748–54.
27. Klein H, Auricchio A, Reek S, Geller C. New primary prevention trials of sudden cardiac death in patients with left ventricular dysfunction: SCD-HeFT and MADIT-II. Am J Cardiol 1999; 83(5B): 91D–97D.
28. Baroldi G, Falzi G, Mariani F. Sudden coronary death: a post-mortem study in 208 selected cases compared to 97 'control' subjects. Am Heart J 1979; 98: 20–31.
29. Packer M. Sudden unexpected death in patients with congestive heart failure: a second frontier. Circulation 1985; 72: 681–5.
30. Cobb LA, Weaver WD. Exercise: a risk for sudden death in patients with coronary artery disease. J Am Coll Cardiol 1986; 7: 215–19.
31. Salerno JA, Previtali M, Chimienti M, Klersy C, Bobba P. Vasospasm and ventricular arrhythmias. Ann N Y Acad Sci 1984; 427: 222–33.
32. Myerburg RJ, Kessler KM, Malloon SM et al. Life-threatening ventricular arrhythmias in patients with silent myocardial ischemia due to coronary artery spasm. N Engl J Med 1992; 326(22): 1451–5.
33. MacAlpin RN. Relation of coronary arterial spasm to sites of organic stenosis. Am J Cardiol 1980; 46: 143–53.
34. Robertson D, Robertson RM, Nies AS et al. Variant angina pectoris: investigation of indexes of sympathetic nervous system function. Am J Cardiol 1979; 43: 1080–5.
35. Buda AJ, Fowles RE, Schroeder JS et al. Coronary artery spasm in the denervated transplanted human heart. A clue to underlying mechanisms. Am J Med 1981; 70(5): 1144–9.
36. Hammon JW, Oates JA. Interaction of platelets with the vessel wall in the pathophysiology of sudden cardiac death. Circulation 1986; 73(2): 224–6.
37. Davies MJ, Thomas A. Thrombosis and acute coronary artery lesions in sudden cardiac ischemic death. N Engl J Med 1984; 310(18): 1137–40.
38. Myerburg RJ, Kessler KM, Zaman L et al. Survivors of prehospital cardiac arrest. JAMA 1982; 247(10): 1485–90.
39. Surawicz B. Ventricular fibrillation. J Am Coll Cardiol 1985; 5(6 Suppl): 43B–54B.
40. Cameron JS, Myerburg RJ, Wong SS et al. Electrophysiologic consequences of chronic experimentally induced left ventricular pressure overload. J Am Coll Cardiol 1983; 2(3): 481–7.

41. Myerburg RJ, Bassett AL, Epstein K et al. Electrophysiologic effects of procainamide in acute and healed experimental ischemic injury of cat myocardium. Circ Res 1982; 50(3): 386–93.
42. Janse MJ, Kleber AG. Electrophysiological changes and ventricular arrhythmias in the early phase of regional myocardial ischemia. Circ Res 1981; 49(5): 1069–81.
43. Salerno JA, Klersy C, Previtali M et al. Correlation between ventricular arrhythmias and occlusion and reperfusion phases in vasosplastic angina pectoris. Acta Med Rom 1983; 21: 309–13.
44. Manning AS, Hearse DJ. Reperfusion-induced arrhythmias: mechanisms and prevention. J Mol Cell Cardiol 1984; 16: 497–518.
45. Gauduel Y, Duvelleroy M. Role of oxygen radicals in cardiac injury due to reoxygenation. J Mol Cell Cardiol 1984; 16: 459–70.
46. Kimura S, Bassett AL, Kohya T et al. Simultaneous recording of action potentials from endocardium and epicardium during ischemia in the isolated cat ventricle: relation of temporal electrophysiological heterogeneities to arrhythmias. Circulation 1986; 74(2): 401–9.
47. Verrier RL, Hagestad EL. Role of the autonomic neuron system in sudden death. In: Josephson ME, ed. Sudden Cardiac Death. Philadelphia: FA Davis, 1985: 41–63.
48. Vassalle M. On the mechanisms underlying cardiac standstill: factors determining success or failure of escape pacemakers in the heart. J Am Coll Cardiol 1985; 5(6 Suppl): 35B–42B.
49. Fozzard HA. Electromechanical dissociation and its possible role in sudden cardiac death. J Am Coll Cardiol 1985; 5(6 Suppl): 31B–34B.
50. Baum RS, Alvarez H, Cobb LA. Survival after resuscitation from out-of-hospital ventricular fibrillation. Circulation 1974; 50(6): 1231–5.
51. Liberthson RR, Nagel EL, Hirschman JC, Nussenfeld SR. Prehospital ventricular fibrillation: prognosis and follow-up course. N Engl J Med 1974; 291(7): 317–21.
52. Fulton M, Lutz W, Donald KW et al. Natural history of unstable angina. Lancet 1972; 1(7756): 860–5.
53. Buxton AE. The primary prevention of sudden cardiac death: prospective identification of the problem. Noninvasive and invasive techniques for risk stratification. In: Dunbar SB, Ellenbogen K, Epstein AE, eds. Sudden Cardiac Death: Past, Present and Future. New York: Futura, 1997: 119–47.
54. Bayes de Luna A, Coumel P, Leclercq JF. Ambulatory sudden death: mechanisms of production of fatal arrhythmia on the basis of data from 157 cases. Am Heart J 1989; 117(1): 151–9.
55. Furukawa T, Rozansky JJ, Nogami J et al. Time-dependent risk of and predictors for cardiac arrest recurrence in survivors of out-of-hospital cardiac arrest with chronic coronary artery disease. Circulation 1989; 80(3): 599–608.

# 2

# Sudden cardiac death: the size of the problem

Alessandro Capucci and Daniela Aschieri

Sudden cardiac death (SCD) is the result of an unresuscitated cardiac arrest, which may be caused by almost all known heart diseases. Most cardiac arrests are due to rapid and/or chaotic activity of the heart (ventricular tachycardia or fibrillation); some are due to extreme slowing of the heart (bradyarrhythmia). These events are called life-threatening arrhythmia and cause sudden death.

The term *massive heart attack,* commonly used in the media to describe sudden death, only infrequently is responsible for SCD. *Heart attack* more properly refers to death of heart muscle tissue due to the loss of blood supply. While a heart attack may cause cardiac arrest and SCD, the terms are not synonymous.

The current definition of SCD describes death within 1 h of onset of symptoms. From a practical point of view, it is very difficult to estimate the duration of symptoms that preceded death among patients found 'dead on arrival'. It is often difficult to obtain information about timing of events and symptoms, in many out-of-hospital cardiac arrest victims. Moreover, many patients may die at home without emergency medical intervention, so obscuring the full extent of the problem. For this reason, it is difficult to establish the real incidence of SCD.

## CARDIOVASCULAR DISEASE: EPIDEMIOLOGIC DATA

Cardiovascular death is considered the main killer in the USA and other western countries. Since 1970, coronary artery disease rates have fallen in general across western Europe and in the USA;[1] nevertheless, the percentage of SCD has increased from 38% to 47%.[2] In fact, even if the age-adjusted rate for cardiovascular disease has been progressively decreasing, in 2001, cardiovascular disease was the main cause of death in the USA, representing the primary cause of death in 931 000 patients, and the secondary cause of death in 477 000 cases. Epidemiologic data show that 39% of all-cause mortality is a cardiovascular disease, thus representing the main cause of death worldwide.[3] Meanwhile, in the USA, cardiovascular disease is progressively decreasing; however, in other European and Asiatic countries, it is increasing with industrialization.[4] It has been calculated that every newborn child has a 47% probability of dying from cardiovascular disease, and it has been estimated that if it were possible to eliminate all cardiovascular disease, the mean expectancy of life should increase by about 7 years. Every year in the USA coronary artery disease causes:[5]

- 502 000 deaths, 185 000 being due to myocardial infarction
- 1.2 million myocardial infarctions (700 000 new myocardial infarctions every year)
- 133 billion dollars spent.

Actually, 13.2 million individuals in USA are affected by symptomatic cardiovascular disease (6.5 million men, 6.7 million women). Asymptomatic cardiovascular diseases are considered to be much more frequent.

It has been calculated that, by 2020, coronary artery disease will be the main cause of death in the world.[1] Autopsy studies on patients that died from traumatic death have demonstrated that arteriosclerosis is still present in children and young persons: coronary disease has been found in 50–75% of young men, of whom 5–10% had significant stenosis. More than 75% of older individuals presented significant coronary disease.[6]

This may help us to understand why SCD may represent in more than 50% of cases the first sign of a coronary asymptomatic artery disease.

Unpublished data from the Division of Adult and Community Health, National Center for Chronic Disease Prevention and Health Promotion, based on demographic data (e.g., age and race/ethnicity) listed on death certificates reported by funeral directors, usually from information provided by the family of the decedent, SCD was defined as death from cardiac disease that occurred out-of-hospital or in an emergency department, or one in which the decedent was reported to be 'dead on arrival' at a hospital. Among 728 743 cardiac disease deaths that occurred in 1999, a total of 462 340 (63.4%) were SCD, 120 244 (16.5%) occurred in an emergency department or were dead on arrival, and 341 780 (46.9%) occurred out-of-hospital. Women had a higher total number of cardiac deaths and higher proportion of out-of-hospital cardiac deaths than men (51.9% of 375 243 and 41.7% of 353 500, respectively), and men had a higher proportion of cardiac deaths that occurred in an emergency department or were dead on arrival (21.2% of 353 500 and 12.0% of 375 243, respectively) (Table 2.1). SCD accounted for 10 460 (75.4%) of all 13 873 cardiac disease deaths in persons aged 35–44 years, and the proportion of cardiac deaths that occurred out-of-hospital increased with age, from 5.8% in persons aged 0–4 years to 61.0% in persons aged ≥85 years. SCD accounted for 63.7% of all cardiac deaths among whites, 62.3% among blacks, 59.8% among Native Americans/Inuits, 55.8% among Asians/Pacific Islanders, and 54.2% among Hispanics. Whites had the highest proportion of cardiac deaths out-of-hospital, and blacks had the highest proportion of cardiac deaths in an emergency department or dead on arrival. The age-adjusted SCD rate was 47.0% higher among men than women (206.5 and 140.7 per 100 000 population, respectively). Blacks had the highest age-adjusted rates (253.6 in men and 175.3 in women) followed by whites (204.5 in men and 138.4 in women), Native Americans/Inuits (132.7 in men and 76.6 in women), and Asians/Pacific Islanders (111.5 in men and 66.5 in women). Non-Hispanics (217.8 in men and 147.3 in women) had higher age-adjusted SCD rates than Hispanics (118.5 in men and 147.3 in women).

## Epidemiologic studies on SCD

SCD is a very common problem that accounts for about 50% of cardiovascular mortality in developed countries.[7–9] The majority of coronary artery disease deaths occur outside the hospital with the largest component as SCD.[10] Although the absolute number of SCD has decreased in parallel with a reduction in overall cardiovascular mortality,[11] the proportion of all cardiovascular deaths that are sudden and unexpected remains constant at approximately 50%.[2,3,12] Epidemiologic studies that have used prospective collection of autopsy reports, emergency medical reports, and medical records to determine the incidence of SCD seem to be more accurate

**Table 2.1** Sudden death in the USA: epidemiologic data per year

| **Overall incidence in adult population** | **300 000** |
|---|---|
| High-coronary-risk subgroup | 220 000 |
| Any prior coronary event | 180 000 |
| EF (ejection fraction) < 30% heart failure | 130 000 |
| Out-of-hospital cardiac arrest survivors | 40 000 |
| Convalescent phase VT/VF after myocardial infarction | 20 000 |

VT/VF: ventricular tachycardia/ventricular fibrillation.
EF: ejection fraction

than studies based on retrospective evaluation of death certifications, which can overestimate SCD incidence[13] due to superficial diagnosis of death at the act of compilation of death certificates.

In the prospective combined Albany-Framingham study of 4120 males, sudden death was observed in 109/234 coronary artery deaths/1000 inhabitants. This means that 47% of deaths are sudden and unexpected. This percentage represents the prevalence of sudden death in a population at high risk of coronary disease, as in the USA.

The annual incidence of SCD has been reported to range from 36 to 128 per 100 000 inhabitants in the study of Becker et al,[14] which used emergency medical system patient reports as the data source. The task force on SCD of the European Society of Cardiology states that the incidence of SCD ranges between 26 and 128/100 000 per year, while the Maastricht[15] study observed an overall incidence of SCD of 97/100 000. This is a population-based study that monitored all cases of out-of-hospital cardiac arrest occurring in victims between 20 and 75 years of age. An overall yearly incidence of SCD of 1 per 1000 was recorded. Overall, 21% of all deaths were sudden and unexpected in men; 14.5% were so in women. Eighty percent of out-of-hospital cases occurred at home and about 15% on the street or in a public place. Forty percent of SCD was unwitnessed. Myerburg and colleagues[16] reviewed the issue of the risk of SCD in population subgroups, and its contribution to the overall burden of SCD. Based on a figure of 300 000 SCD/annum in the USA the population incidence was just over 1/1000 inhabitants per year. In the Italian city of Piacenza (250 000 inhabitants), the estimated incidence of SCD from emergency medical reports is 1.2/1000 inhabitants.[17]

## Incidence and absolute number of sudden death

More than 300 000 SCD occur annually among the unselected adult population in the USA[18] with an overall incidence of 0.1–0.2% per year. This calculation includes the 20–25% of SCD victims whose cardiac arrest is the first clinical manifestation of previously silent or unrecognized heart disease[19–21] plus those with various degrees of increased risk identified by established clinical characteristics or risk-factor profiles. When the very-high-risk subgroups are removed from this population base, the calculated incidence for the remaining patients obviously decreases, but represents the majority of the events because of the larger size of the population. In Figure 2.1, the magnitude of the risk, expressed as incidence, is compared with the total number of events per year. The absolute number of deaths becomes

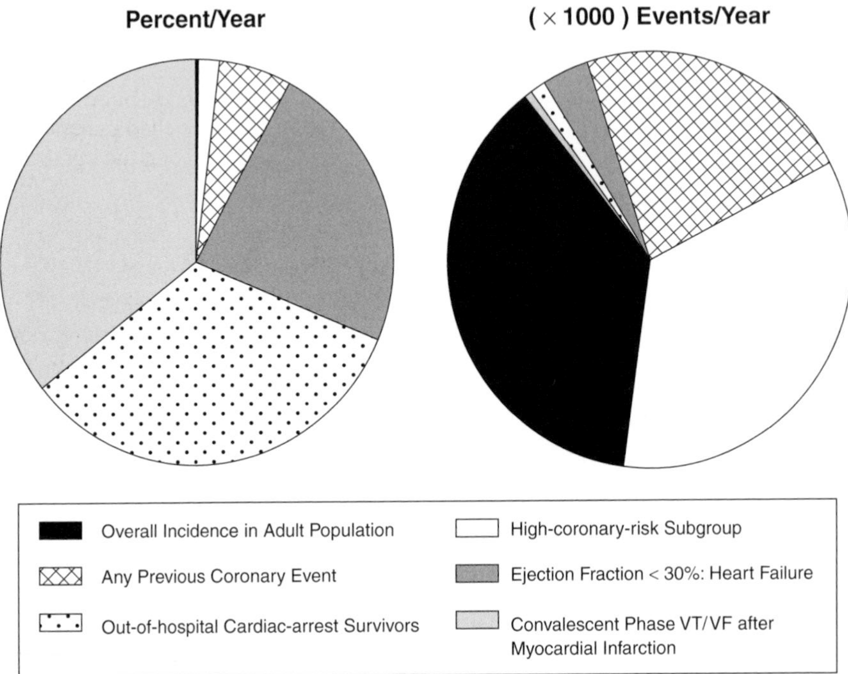


**Figure 2.1** SCD among population subgroups. Estimates of incidence (percent per year) and total number of SCD per year are shown for the overall adult population in the USA and for higher-risk subgroups. The overall estimated incidence is 0.1–0.2% per year, totaling more than 300 000 deaths per year. Within subgroups identified by increasing risk factors, the increasing incidence is accompanied by progressively decreasing total numbers. VT/VF: ventricular tachycardia-ventricular fibrillation.

progressively smaller as the subgroups become more focused, limiting the impact of interventions to the much smaller subgroups.

## SUDDEN DEATH: IS IT THE BEST DEATH?

Sudden death is, philosophically considered, 'the best death', due to its rapid nature with no pain or long-term suffering. One of the particular aspects of sudden death is the abrupt onset of the event. The initial rhythm for most SCD is ventricular fibrillation.[22] This is the more shocking aspect for the public and the community, leaving public opinion uncertain on this event. Some studies have evaluated the potential risk to public safety of sudden death. Myerburg et al[23] reported data from an observational study of 1348 sudden deaths caused by coronary artery disease in people older than 65 years of age during a period of 7 years. In this study, 7.5% of people were engaged in activity at the time of death that was potentially dangerous to others: 56 were driving public or private cars, 15 were driving trucks, 10 were working at altitude, and two were piloting aircraft, and 9.1% were in situations which could potentially be dangerous due to their work: 57 taxi and truck drivers, eight aircraft pilots, nine bus drivers, and nine policemen and firemen. No catastrophic events resulted from these cardiac arrests but only minor damage. Several other studies have led to the conclusion that the risk to the community is small.[24] However, it may not be considered the best death. Long-term survival among patients who have undergone rapid defibrillation after out-of-hospital cardiac arrest is similar to that among age-, sex-, and disease-matched patients who did not have out-of-hospital cardiac arrest. The quality of life among the majority of survivors is similar to that of the general population.[25]

## RISK FACTORS ASSOCIATED WITH SCD

Risk factors generally accepted as associated with heart disease include family history of heart disease, increased age, being male, hypertension, increased blood cholesterol, cigarette smoking, and diabetes. The main three risk factors that increase risk of SCD are history of a previous myocardial infarction, depressed left ventricular ejection fraction, and presence of complex ventricular ectopy.[26]

### Family history

Familial SCD is frequently associated with a specific syndrome such as long-QT syndrome, hypertrophic cardiomyopathy, and familial SCD in infants and children. Obviously, hereditary coronary artery disease places some families more at risk of sudden death.

### Age

Incidence of SCD occurring out-of-hospital varies with age, gender, and presence or absence of history of cardiovascular disease. In men 60–69 years of age with prior history of heart disease, SCD rates as high as 8 per 1000 per year have been reported.[27]

### Gender

The male:female ratio for SCD was 75–89% in three prospective studies of out-of-hospital cardiac arrest.[28–30] In the Framingham study, the excess risk in men was 6.7:1 in the 55–64-year age group and 2.1:1 in the 65–74-year age group. In the 20-year follow-up, the Framingham study demonstrated a 3.8-fold increased incidence in men compared to women.[31]

### Race

Studies comparing racial differences and risk of SCD in whites and blacks with coronary artery disease have yielded inconclusive data.[32] Interplay between race and cultural factors may operate in SCD in populations originally at low risk of SCD.[33]

### SCD after a cardiac event: time dependence of events

In patients with previous diagnosed cardiovascular disease, there is a time-dependence-increased risk of sudden death after major cardiovascular events compared to patients with no major events.[34] The events that expose patients to major risk of sudden death are myocardial infarction, episodes of heart failure or sudden cardiac arrest. This risk is higher during the first 6–18 months after one of these events, as shown in Figure 2.2. After 18–24 months, the risk pattern of sudden death declines.

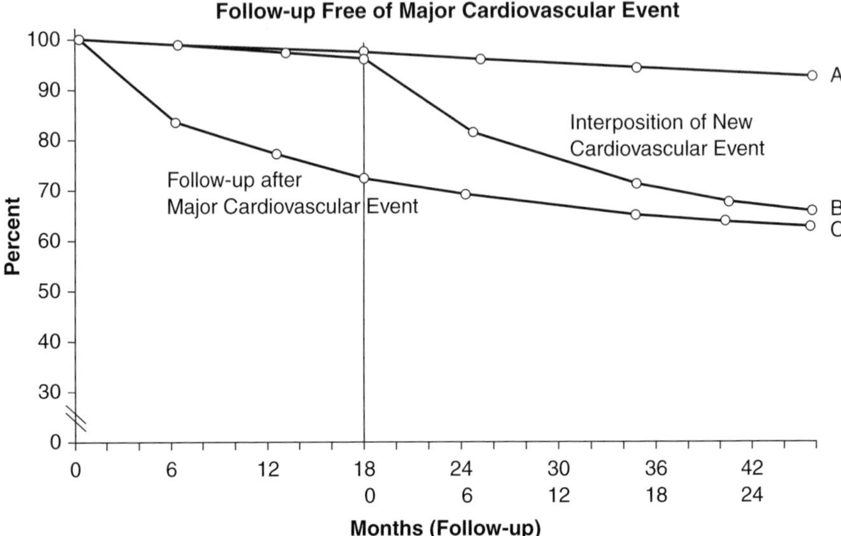


**Figure 2.2** Time-dependence of risk after cardiovascular events. Survival curves for hypothetical patients with known cardiovascular disease free of a major index event (curve A) and for patients surviving major cardiovascular events (curve C). Attrition is accelerated during the initial 6–24 months after the event. Curve B shows the dynamics of risk over time in low-risk patients with an interposed major event that is normalized to a time point (for example, 18 months). The subsequent attrition is accelerated for 6–24 months.[34]

## Myocardial infarction

The risk of sudden death after surviving a heart attack is highest for certain patients in the first 30 days and then declines. Survival during 3 years after an acute myocardial infarction is a function of ejection fraction (EF), as represented in Figure 2.3. The greatest change of risk is in patients with an EF of 30–40%.[35] An EF equal to or less than 30% is the single most important predictor of sudden death, even if it is a parameter with low specificity. A higher number of premature ventricular beats also increases the risk of sudden death. In particular, the presence of left ventricular dysfunction appears to exert its influence more strongly in the first 6 months after myocardial infarction, as shown in Figure 2.3 (curves C and D). Data from recent studies[36,37] have shown 5% and 2%, respectively, incidences of sudden death at 2–5 year follow-up after acute myocardial infarction.

The risk of sudden death is highest in the first 30 days after myocardial infarction among patients with left ventricular dysfunction, heart failure, or both.[38] This is also the result of a recent secondary analysis of a study evaluating the effects of two drugs used for blood pressure control and heart failure (valsartan and captopril) in 14 609 subjects with myocardial infarction complicated by heart failure, left ventricular dysfunction (EF of 40% or less), or both. About 4000 subjects had an EF of 30% or less, 5000 had an EF of 31–40% and 2400 had an EF of >40%. For the first 30 days after myocardial infarction, the rate of sudden death was 1.4% per month (14/1000 persons during the month). This progressively declined over time with a rate of 0.18% per month (18/10 000 persons per month) during the second year after

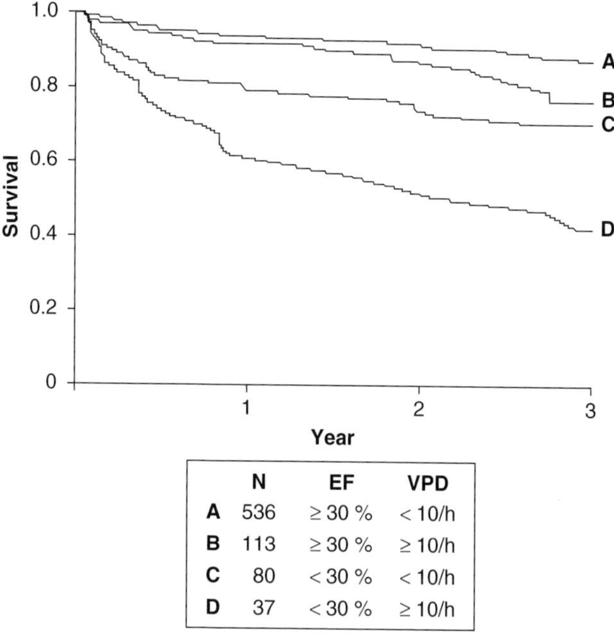


| | N | EF | VPD |
|---|---|---|---|
| A | 536 | ≥ 30 % | < 10/h |
| B | 113 | ≥ 30 % | ≥ 10/h |
| C | 80 | < 30 % | < 10/h |
| D | 37 | < 30 % | ≥ 10/h |

**Figure 2.3** Kaplan–Meier estimates representing 3-year follow-up after acute myocardial infarction. The frequency of both ventricular premature depolarization (VPD) and depressed ejection fractions (EF) contributes to increasing mortality rates. As risk increases by presence of neither (curve A), one (curves B and C), or both (curve D) of these predictors, increasing risk is expressed preferentially within the first year (curves C and D).[45]

myocardial infarction and 0.14% per month during the third year. Even in this study, the risk of sudden death was correlated with EF. During the first 30 days after myocardial infarction, the rate was 2.3% per month in those with EF of <30% compared to about 0.9% per month in those with EF of >30%. Nineteen percent of all sudden deaths or episodes of cardiac arrest with resuscitation occurred within the first 30 days after myocardial infarction, and 83% of all patients who died suddenly did so in the first 30 days after hospital discharge. Each decrease of 5 percentage points in the left ventricular EF was associated with a 21% adjusted increase in the risk of sudden death or cardiac arrest with resuscitation in the first 30 days.

This study is important because it describes the risk of sudden death after myocardial infarction in the new era of treatment with reperfusion therapy (with fibrinolytic and other drugs or mechanically by cardiac catheterization) and more aggressive use of beta-blockers. It reaffirms that sudden death is a significant threat even among stable patients and those with EF of >40% who have clinical heart failure, and that the greatest risk is during the first month after infarction.

What is the practical implication of these epidemiologic data? Clearly, there is a real and significant risk of sudden death after an acute cardiac event and it is highest during the first month, with progressive decrease until about 1 year when the risk stabilizes at about 0.15% per month (about 1.8% per year). This property of risk must be integrated into strategies designed to intervene in such patients.

## SCD in heart failure

SCD is an important cause of death in heart failure, regardless of its etiology. As the severity of heart failure progresses from New York Heart Association functional class II to IV, the annual mortality increases from about 10% to 50%. The proportion of these deaths that are sudden decreases from about 65% in class II heart failure to about 20% in class IV heart failure. Kjekshus[39] analyzed a group of studies of heart-failure-related deaths, contrasting the probability of death and the ratio of sudden to total deaths as they relate to functional classification. In studies in which the mean functional class was between class I and class II, the overall death rate was relatively low, but 67% of the deaths were sudden. In contrast, among studies with mean functional classifications close to class IV, the overall death rate was high, but the fraction of sudden deaths was only 29%. In the former circumstance, a therapeutic intervention targeted on all-cause mortality would be less efficient (that is, only a small fraction of the total population exposed to the intervention would have the potential to benefit from it), whereas, for the latter, efficiency would be high. For an intervention specific to the problem of SCD, however, efficiency in the former case would be relatively high (67% of all deaths are sudden), whereas for the latter, efficiency for SCD would be low because of the dominance of nonsudden deaths. Although the majority of these sudden deaths are due to ventricular tachyarrhythmia, bradyarrhythmia and pulseless electrical activity (PEA), formally known as electromechanical dissociation (EMD), have also been noted at the time of SCD in hospitalized patients who were not in pulmonary edema or cardiogenic shock prior to collapse.

## Recurrence of SCD

In the pre-ICD era, studies from Seattle[40] and Miami[41] indicated that the risk of recurrent sudden death after a first resuscitated cardiac arrest was about 30% at 1 year and 45% at 2 years. This may be considered the natural history of survivors of a sudden cardiac arrest treated with medical therapy in the early 1970s.

Moreover, the risk of recurrent cardiac arrest in patients with hypertrophic cardiomyopathy was lower (33%) in a mean follow-up of 7 years.[42] In the report of Furukava et al,[43] 101 consecutive patients with chronic coronary artery disease who had survived out-of-hospital cardiac arrest in the absence of acute myocardial infarction were followed prospectively. During a mean follow-up of 27 months, cardiac arrest recurred in 21 patients. The actuarial rate of cardiac arrest recurrence was 11.2% during the first 6 months of follow-up ('high-risk early phase') and then decreased to less than 4% in each subsequent 6-month period. Cox multivariate proportional hazards analysis identified an EF of $<35\%$ ($P=0.0013$) and persistent inducibility of ventricular tachyarrhythmia ($P=0.0025$) as independent predictors of cardiac arrest recurrence for the entire follow-up period (Figure 2.4).

## Sudden death and athletes

SCD in athletes, although relatively uncommon, is a well-recognized condition generally associated with some congenital abnormalities. However, it continues to be of vast interest to the public, as athletes are seen as a distinct group able to tolerate more intense physical activity than the general population. Obviously, intense activity predisposes susceptible athletes to SCD; hence the importance of pre-participation screening tests. Maron et al[44] utilized insurance program data for high-school

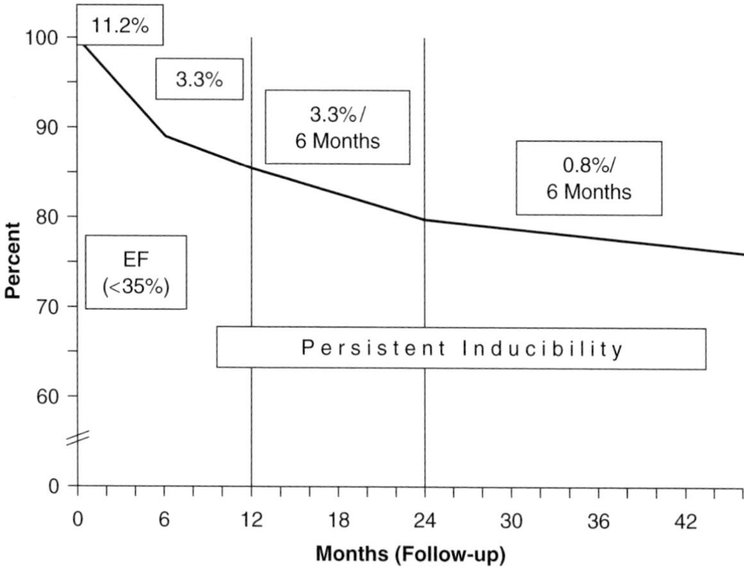


**Figure 2.4** Survival curve showing time-dependence of risk for recurrence among survivors of cardiac arrest. The risk was highest during the first 6 months.[34]

athletes in Minnesota to calculate prevalence rates during the 12-year period from 1985 to 1997 for athletes in grades 10–12. A total of 651 695 athletes competed in 27 sports for a total of 1 453 280 overall participations. Three deaths occurred from anomalous origin of the left coronary artery from the right sinus of Valsalva, congenital aortic stenosis and myocarditis. The calculated risk of sudden death was 1:500 000 participations. The annual rate of sudden death was 0.46/100 000 participants. Thiene et al[45] assessed the prevalence of sudden death in young athletes in the Veneto region of Italy: they calculated an annual rate of 0.75/100 000 nonathletes, annual rate of 1.6/100 000 athletes.

## CONCLUSION

The proportion of SCD that occur out-of-hospital has increased since 1989.[46] Death and disability from a heart attack can be reduced if persons having a heart attack can immediately recognize its symptoms and call 911 for emergency care. These symptoms are chest discomfort or pain; pain or discomfort in one or both arms or in the back, neck, jaw, or stomach; and shortness of breath. Other symptoms are breaking out in a cold sweat, nausea, and light-headedness. Prevention of the first cardiac event through risk factor reduction (e.g., tobacco control, weight management, physical activity, and control of high blood pressure and cholesterol intake) should continue to be the focus of public health efforts to reduce the number of deaths from heart disease. Education and systems support to promote physician adherence to clinical practice guidelines and more timely access to emergency cardiac care also are important in the prevention and early treatment of a heart attack. Prehospital emergency medical service systems can assist in reducing SCD rates by dispatching appropriately trained and properly equipped response personnel as rapidly as possible in the event of cardiac emergencies. However, national efforts are needed to increase the proportion of the public that can recognize and respond to symptoms and can intervene when someone is having a heart attack, including calling 911, attempting cardiac resuscitation, and using automated external defibrillators until emergency personnel arrive.

## REFERENCES


1. Sans S, Kesteloot H, Kromhout D. The burden of cardiovascular diseases mortality in Europe. Task Force of the European Society of Cardiology on Cardiovascular Mortality and Morbidity Statistics in Europe. Eur Heart J 1997; 18(12): 1231–48.
2. Josephson M, Wellens HJ. Implantable defibrillators and sudden cardiac death. Circulation 2004; 109(22): 2685–91.
3. Murray CJ, Lopez AD. Alternative projections of mortality and disability by cause 1990–2020: Global Burden of Disease Study. Lancet 1997; 349: 1498–504.
4. Reddy KS, Yusuf S. Emerging epidemic of cardiovascular disease in developing countries. Circulation 1998; 97: 596–601.
5. American Heart Association. Heart and stroke statistics – 2004 update. www.americanheart.org.
6. Berenson GS, Srinivasan SR, Bao W et al. Association between multiple cardiovascular risk factors and atherosclerosis in children and young adults. The Bogalusa Heart Study. N Engl J Med 1998; 338: 1650–6.
7. Myerburg RJ, Kessler KM, Castellanos A. Sudden cardiac death. Structure, function, and time-dependence of risk. Circulation 1992; 85(Suppl 1): 2–10.
8. Gillum RF. Sudden coronary death in the United States: 1980–1985. Circulation 1989; 79: 756–65.
9. de Lorgeril M, Salen P, Defaye P et al. Dietary prevention of sudden cardiac death. Eur Heart J 2002; 23: 277–85.
10. Fox CS, Evans JC, Larson MG et al. Temporal trends in coronary heart disease mortality and sudden cardiac death from 1950 to 1999: the Framingham Heart Study. Circulation 2004; 110: 522–7.
11. Epstein FH, Pisa Z. International comparisons in ischemic heart disease mortality. Proceedings of the Conference on the Decline in Coronary Heart Disease Mortality. NIH Publication no. 79-1610. Washington, DC: US Government Printing Office, 1979: 58–88.
12. Myerburg RJ, Castellanos A. Cardiac arrest and sudden cardiac death. In: Braunwald E, ed. Heart Disease: A Textbook of Cardiovascular Medicine. 4th edn. Philadelphia: WB Saunders, 1992: 756–89.
13. Chung SS, Jui J, Gunson K et al. Current burden of sudden cardiac death: multiple source surveillance versus retrospective death certificate-based review in a large US community. J Am Coll Cardiol 2004; 44: 1268–75.
14. Becker LB, Smith DW, Rhodes KV. Incidence of cardiac arrest: a neglected factor in evaluating survival rates. Ann Emerg Med 1993; 22(1): 86–91.
15. Vreede-Swagemakers JJ, Gorgels AP, Dobois-Arbouw WI et al. Out-of-hospital cardiac arrest in the 1990's: a population-based study in the Maastricht area on incidence, characteristics, and survival. J Am Coll Cardiol 1997; 30; 1500–5.
16. Myerburg RJ, Kessler KM, Castellanos A. Sudden cardiac death. Structure, function, and time dependence of risk. Circulation 1992; 85: 2–10.
17. Podrid PJ, Myerburg RJ. Epidemiology and stratification of risk for sudden cardiac death. Clin Cardiol 2005; 28(11 Suppl 1): 3–11.
18. Report of the Working Group on Arteriosclerosis of the National Heart, Lung, and Blood Institute. Vol 2. Patient Oriented Research – Fundamental and Applied, Sudden Cardiac Death. NIH Publication no. 83-2035. Washington, DC: US Government Printing Office, 1981: 114–22.

19. Kannel WB, Doyle JT, McNamara PM, Quickenton P, Gordon T. Precursors of sudden coronary death. Factors related to the incidence of sudden death. Circulation 1979; 51: 606–13.
20. Kuller LH. Sudden death – definition and epidemiologic considerations. Prog Cardiovasc Dis 1980; 23: 1–12.
21. Goldstein S. The necessity of a uniform definition of sudden coronary death: witnessed death within 1 hour of the onset of acute symptoms. Am Heart J 1982; 103: 156–9.
22. Demirovic J, Myerburg RJ. Epidemiology of sudden coronary death: an overview. Prog Cardiovasc Dis 1994; 37(1): 39–48.
23. Myerburg RJ, Davis JH. The medical ecology of public safety. I. Sudden death due to coronary artery disease. Am Heart J 1964; 68: 586–95.
24. Kervin AJ. Sudden death while driving. Can Med Assoc J 1984; 1321: 312–4.
25. Bunch TJ, White RD, Gersh BJ et al. Long-term outcomes of out-of-hospital cardiac arrest after successful early defibrillation. N Engl J Med 2003; 348(26): 2626–33.
26. Fogoros RN. Electrophysiologic Testing. 2nd edn. Cambridge, MA: Blackwell Science, 1995.
27. Sans S, Kesteloot H, Kromhout D. The burden of cardiovascular diseases mortality in Europe. Task Force of the European Society of Cardiology on Cardiovascular Mortality and Morbidity Statistics in Europe. Eur Heart J 1997; 18: 1231–48.
28. Liberthson RR, Nagel EL, Hirschman JC, Nussenfeld SR. Prehospital ventricular fibrillation: prognosis and follow up courses. N Engl J Med 1974; 317(291): 1231–5.
29. Baum RS, Alvarez H, Cobb LA. Survival after resuscitation from out of hospital cardiac arrest. Circulation 1974; 1231(50): 24–31.
30. James TN, MacLean WAH. Paroxysmal ventricular arrhythmias and familial sudden cardiac death associated with neural lesions in the heart. Chest 1980; 78(24): 3–21.
31. Kannel WB, Thomas HE. Sudden coronary death: the Framingham study. Ann N Y Acad Sci 1982; 382(3): 155–75.
32. Goldstein S. Sudden Death and Coronary Artery Disease. Mckisco, N Y: Futura 1974.
33. Robertson TL, Kato H, Gordon T et al. Epidemiologic studies of coronary heart disease and stroke in Japanese men living in Japan, Hawaii and California. Coronary heart disease risk factors in Japan and Hawaii. Am J Cardiol 1977; 39(2): 244–9.
34. Myerburg RJ, Kessler KM, Castellanos A. Sudden cardiac death. Structure, function, and time-dependence of risk. Circulation 1992; 85(Suppl 1): 2–10.
35. Bigger JT Jr. Antiarrhythmic therapy: an overview. Am J Cardiol 1984; 53: 8B–16B.
36. Farb A, Tang AL, Burke AP et al. Sudden coronary death. Frequency of active coronary lesions, inactive coronary lesions, and myocardial infarction. Circulation 1995; 92: 1701–9.
37. Patterson E, Holland K, Eller BT, Lucchesi BR. Ventricular fibrillation resulting from ischemia at a site remote from previous myocardial infarction. A conscious canine model of sudden coronary death. Am J Cardiol 1982; 50: 1414–23.
38. Solomon S, Zelenkofske S, McMurray SSV et al. Sudden death in patients with myocardial infarction and left ventricular dysfunction, heart failure or both. N Engl J Med 2005; 352(25): 2581–8.
39. Bigger JT Jr. Relation between left ventricular dysfunction and ventricular arrhythmias after myocardial infarction. Am J Cardiol 1986; 57(3): 8B–14B.
40. Kjekshus J. Arrhythmias and mortality in congestive heart failure. Am J Cardiol 1990; 65: 42I–8I.
41. Baum RS, Alvarez H 3rd, Cobb LA. Survival after resuscitation from out-of-hospital ventricular fibrillation. Circulation 1974; 50(6): 1231–5.
42. Liberthson RR, Nagel EL, Hirschman JC, Nussenfeld SR. Prehospital ventricular defibrillation. Prognosis and follow-up course. N Engl J Med 1974; 291(7): 317–21.
43. Cecchi F, Maron BJ, Epstein SE. Long-term outcome of patients with hypertrophic cardiomyopathy successfully resuscitated after cardiac arrest. J Am Coll Cardiol 1989; 13(6): 1283–8.

44. Furukawa T, Rozanski JJ, Nogami A et al. Time-dependent risk of and predictors for cardiac arrest recurrence in survivors of out-of-hospital cardiac arrest with chronic coronary artery disease. Circulation 1989; 80(3): 599–608.
45. Maron BJ, Gohman TE, Aeppli D. Prevalence of sudden cardiac death during competitive sports activities in Minnesota high school athletes. J Am Coll Cardiol 1998; 32(7): 1881–4.
46. Thiene G, Basso C, Corrado D. Sudden death in the young and in the athlete: causes, mechanisms and prevention. Cardiologia 1999; 44(Suppl 1): 415–21.
47. Zheng Z-J, Croft JB, Giles WH, Mensah GA. Sudden cardiac death in the United States, 1989 to 1998. Circulation 2001; 104: 2158–63.

# 3

# Pathophysiology of sudden death: electrophysiologic mechanism in different clinical conditions

Paolo Della Bella and Stefania Riva

The onset of life-threatening ventricular tachyarrhythmia or severe bradycardia, asystole or pulseless electrical activity (electromechanical dissociation (EMD)) is the final result of a cascade of events that involves interaction between anatomic and functional substrates and a triggering event that leads to sudden cardiac death (SCD)[1,2] (Figure 3.1).

Structural abnormalities of the myocardium, coronary arteries, or cardiac nerves or gene abnormalities provide the substrate on which a transient initiating event acts. The vast majority of cardiac arrest episodes occur in patients with structural abnormalities and coronary artery disease seems to be responsible for almost 75% of all SCD.[3] An acute transmural myocardial infarction is present, however, in only 20% of the cases, and it is assumed that transient myocardial ischemia, caused, for example, by unstable platelet thrombi or coronary spasm, plays a major role as transient precipitating factor.[4] Congestive heart failure, myocardial hypertrophy and regional autonomic dysfunction may also be important.[5] However, sudden, predominantly arrhythmic cardiac deaths also occur in apparently healthy individuals, usually unexpectedly.[6]

SCD due to severe bradyarrhythmia represents nearly 15% of all the cases; it occurs more commonly in severely diseased hearts, in the setting of end-stage heart failure, and represents an irreversible form of EMD.[7] The outlook for patients presenting bradycardia, asystole or EMD at the time of cardiac arrest is worse than for patients exhibiting ventricular tachycardia (VT) or ventricular fibrillation (VF).

The electrophysiologic mechanism underlying cardiac arrest due to severe bradyarrhythmia is the inability of subsidiary pacemaker cells of the heart to generate impulse from lack of sinus-node or atrioventricular node activity, or the failure of a spontaneous impulse to propagate and activate the heart; all of these are generally consequences of diffuse involvement of subendocardial Purkinje fibers.[8] Different mechanisms may result in the suppression of automaticity or the prevention of impulse propagation: ionic changes in currents that contribute to spontaneous depolarization; intrinsic heart diseases, such as myocardial infarction, infiltrative diseases involving sinus and/or atrioventricular nodes; the action of drugs such as antiarrhythmic agents; changes in neural activity and autonomic balance; and neurally mediated factors linked to, for example, myocardial infarction, aortic stenosis, or congestive heart failure.[9]Pulseless electrical activity (EMD) is characterized by a stable cardiac rhythm in the absence of an effective mechanical contractile function of the heart. It can be subdivided into primary and secondary forms. The former

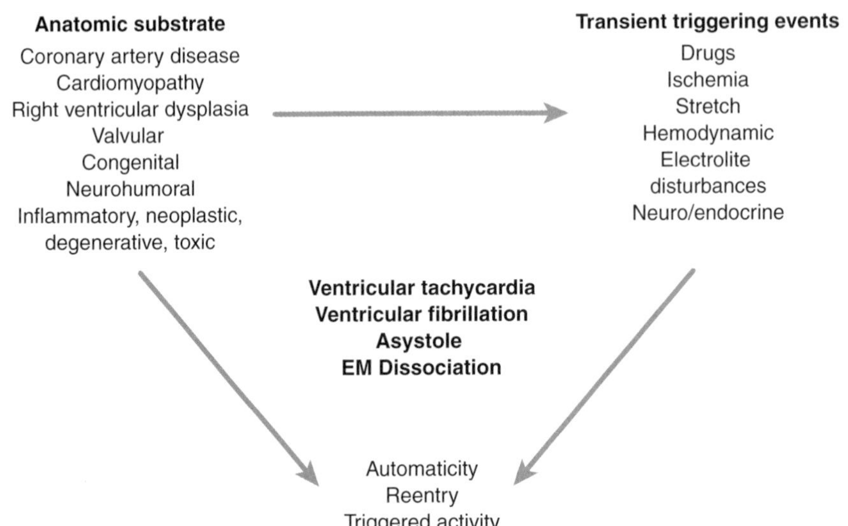


**Figure 3.1** Chain of events leading to sudden cardiac death.

occurs more frequently and is characterized by the inability of a depressed ventricular muscle to contract despite the presence of electrical activity. Usually, it represents the end stage of advanced heart disease, but it can also occur in the setting of extensive myocardial infarction or ischemia, or after cardiac resuscitation.

In the secondary form, cardiac output is severely reduced because of abrupt reduction in preload, mechanical obstruction, but the intrinsic contractile function of the ventricle is normal[10] (Table 3.1).

Most commonly (85%), SCD is caused by life-threatening ventricular tachyarrhythmia; often by the onset of monomorphic VT that degenerates into VF, and, less frequently, by polymorphic VT or VF directly.[11]

VF represents the end of a multitude of disturbances, and the sources of arrhythmogenesis are unlikely to be due to any single abnormality. It can be said that an altered myocardium supports fatal arrhythmia initiated by a transient triggering event. Altered myocardium can be due to scar, hypertrophy, or myocite disorders, but is normally insufficient by itself to produce SCD. Transient perturbations of the balance, crucial to precipitate life-threatening arrhythmia, might include transient myocardial ischemia, platelet and thrombus activation, autonomic nervous system dysfunction, electrolyte disturbance, hypoxemia, acidosis, or abnormalities in gene expression.[1,12,13] Moreover, although many patients have anatomic and functional substrates predisposing to fatal arrhythmia, and many experience triggering precipitating events, only a few patients develop SCD. This fact indicates the role of individual and genetic risk-predisposing factors, the identification of which is now certainly crucial to future effective preventive strategies and could explain the final common molecular mechanism of fatal arrhythmias.[14,15]

The most important electrophysiologic feature promoting VF is electrical heterogeneity; that is, the coexistence in the same myocardium of cells in different stages of repolarization and depolarization and/or the presence of zone-of-conduction

**Table 3.1** Electromechanical dissociation: secondary causes

| |
|---|
| Impaired contractility (myocardial depressant drugs) |
| Increased afterload |
| Aortic or pulmonary stenosis |
| Massive pulmonary embolism |
| Hypertrophic cardiomyopathy |
| Primary pulmonary hypertension |
| Decreased preload |
| Cardiac tamponade |
| Massive hemorrhage |
| Sepsis |
| Mechanical obstruction |
| Intracardiac thrombus |
| Myxoma |
| Prosthetic valve dysfunction |

delay or block. Even a normal heart in a normal state can be in this condition, because different heart cells have different refractoriness, action potential and conduction velocities. Moreover, different pathologic conditions can induce the occurrence of heterogeneity at an extreme degree: for example, ischemia may induce conduction delay and/or block in one region of the heart, and regional sympathetic dysfunction or unequal stretch can produce regional electrophysiologic alterations that can generate re-entry, automaticity or triggered activity, and at last induce VF.[5,16]

The interaction between a triggering event and a susceptible myocardium causes the disorganization of the physiologic model of myocardial activation into uncoordinated, multiple re-entry circuits or wavelets. The length of these circuits is determined by the product of conduction velocity and refractory period; thus, it may vary with the characteristics of the tissue and the factors responsible for the re-entry, such as ischemia, prior infarction, or drugs.[1] Usually, VF is initiated by a premature triggering beat that conducts slowly and inhomogeneously and generates a wavebreak initiating re-entry. The premature beat can result from different mechanisms, such as triggered activity, enhanced automaticity, or re-entry occurring as a result of early or late afterdepolarization.

According to Wiggers et al, VF is characterized by four stages.[17] The first, the tachysystolic or undulatory, lasts a few seconds, correlates with a surface ECG consistent with VT, can be terminated by a second premature beat, and is characterized by a pattern of activation that forms a figure-of-eight re-entry.[18] The second, convulsive uncoordination, correlates with VF on the ECG, lasts 15–40 s, and is characterized by multiple, simultaneous re-entry circuits providing the constant source of activation required to maintain VF.[19] The third stage, lasting 2–3 min, is called tremulous uncoordination and is characterized by a decrease in VF rate, and by an endocardial-epicardial gradient in activation rate.[20] The final stage is that of atonic fibrillation, with complete failure of contractility. The identification of the different stages of VF has relevant clinical implication: stage 1 can be self-terminating; but, once stage 2 is established, electrical defibrillation is the most effective therapy. However, in the majority of cases of out-of-hospital cardiac arrest, the direct-current shocks are delivered when VF is in stage 4; that is, when they are thought to be less effective.

Although it is well known that four stages of VF exist, the mechanisms underlying this fatal arrhythmia still remain incompletely understood. Data collected from animal models developed in recent years have led to two different hypotheses, as VF occurs in the setting of atrial fibrillation: the multiple wavelet hypothesis and the focal source hypothesis.

The first hypothesis assumes that the process of wavebreak, or wave splitting, generates continuously new multiple re-entry circuits, or wavelets, maintaining VF.[21] Wavebreak occurs because of anatomic heterogeneity and nonuniform dispersion of refractoriness. Furthermore, it was shown that even in homogeneous tissue, spiral waves could break, suggesting that dynamically induced heterogeneity, in addition to pre-existing heterogeneity, may play an important role in causing the initial process of wavebreak. Recently, data from the computerized mapping studies of Choi et al[22] and Valderrabano et al[23] have corroborated this hypothesis. They show that during the initial phases of VF, dynamic wavebreak is likely to be very important in maintaining VF. However, as VF proceeds, the heart becomes ischemic, flattening action potential duration restitution and promoting nonuniform regional electrophysiologic heterogeneity.

The focal source or mother rotor hypothesis suggests that the wavebreak may be an epiphenomenon, related to Wenckebach-like conduction, as impulses originating from a relatively stable mother rotor are unable to sustain 1:1 conduction through the surrounding heterogeneous tissue. In this case, the mother rotor, or a rapid firing focal source, rather than wavebreak, is the engine of VF.[24]

The third possibility is that the two hypotheses are complementary and not competitive, crucially suggesting that different types of VF may coexist in the same heart at different times. Wu et al have recently demonstrated that two types of VF coexist in isolated rabbit hearts linked to the electrical restitution properties of the heart.[25]

Type I, or fast, VF is characterized by wandering wavelets and organized re-entry with short life spans. It is associated with steep action potential duration restitution and flat conduction velocity restitution. Slow VF, or type II, is associated with flat action potential duration restitution and broad conduction velocity restitution, and rarely shows wave–wave interaction or epicardial re-entry. Rather, the mapped area always shows a single, long wavefront or a single epicardial breakthrough emerging from the same region repetitively. As this wavefront propagates outward, it frequently developes wavebreaks at some locations, suggesting fibrillatory conduction block.

In summary, although type I VF is more consistent with the multiple wavelet hypothesis, type II suggests the presence of a rapid, focally firing and relatively stable source as the fundamental driver of VF.

Moreover, the findings of Wu et al[25] may partially explain Wiggers' four stages of VF. Wiggers' stage 1 resembles VT that degenerates into multiple wavelets (stage 2), because of a steep action potential duration restitution. Drugs that flatten action potential duration restitution may prevent this degeneration. As ischemia progresses, reduced excitability may convert fast (Wiggers' stage 2) VF into slow (Wiggers' stages 3 and 4) VF.

Two types of VF can thus coexist in the same heart, and, more important, in the clinical setting, type I VF induces acute global ischemia, which flattens action potential duration restitution, decreases excitability, and promotes increased tissue heterogeneity sufficiently to convert it to type II VF.[26] In other words, type I VF normally leads inexorably to type II VF.

In contrast, particularly in patients with structurally normal heart, VF often undergoes spontaneous recovery. Spontaneous defibrillation occurs when type I VF does not convert to lethal type II VF, or type II spontaneously reverts to type I.

Patients with Brugada syndrome, for example, frequently experience repeated aborted SCD as the result of nonsustained or self-defibrillating VF. Acute global ischemia, induced by VF, by flattening action potential duration restitution, may indeed be initially antifibrillatory and help to prevent perpetuation of type I VF, especially in hearts without pre-existing regional ischemia.[27]

Increased myocardial catecholamine content promotes self-defibrillation, probably by delaying the conversion from fast (type I) to slow (type II) VF, or delaying the decrease in excitability during type II VF.[26] The probability of successful defibrillation is increased by epinephrine injection or by chest compressions that improve excitability by restoring coronary blood flow and washing out ischemic metabolites.[28]

## CLINICAL IMPLICATIONS

The elucidation of mechanisms underlying the initiation of serious or fatal ventricular arrhythmia in the human heart remains a major challenge for medical scientists and clinicians and has important clinical implications.

### Radiofrequency catheter ablation of VF

If the mother rotor or focal source hypothesis is correct, catheter ablation of single focus could prevent the triggering of lethal arrhythmia-like VF.

Recently, Haissaguerre et al[29] demonstrated that primary idiopathic VF is characterized by dominant triggers from the distal Purkinje system. In 27 patients resuscitated from recurrent episodes of VF, these foci, with rapid electrical discharges, were successfully eliminated by focal radiofrequency catheter ablation. The authors observed that the patients had, during periods of arrhythmia, isolated premature beats with a morphology identical to those triggering VF. Two groups of arrhythmia origins could be distinguished: one (four cases) originating from right ventricular outflow tract, and one (the majority) from different locations in the Purkinje system. Catheter ablation of these triggers completely eliminated recurrence of VF, as confirmed by implanting cardioverter defibrillator (ICD) interrogation.

More recently, Haissaguerre et al[30] demonstrated the importance of focal triggers in the development of malignant, life-threatening ventricular arrhythmia also in patients with surface ECG abnormalities such as long-QT syndrome and Brugada syndrome. Triggering beats observed in these patients were elicited from the Purkinje system (especially in long-QT syndrome) or from the right ventricular outflow tract (notably in Brugada syndrome). Radiofrequency catheter ablation of these foci abolished premature beats and eliminated malignant arrhythmia.

A similar mechanism has also been described in patients with electrical storm early after myocardial infarction. Bansch et al[31] reported on four patients with incessant VF and VT after myocardial infarction, despite successful reperfusion, amiodarone and beta-blocker therapy. In all four patients, the authors demonstrated that ventricular premature beats with right bundle branch morphology triggered VF or VT. Moreover, radiofrequency catheter ablation of these beats efficiently prevented life-threatening ventricular arrhythmia recurrence. As in Haissaguerre's study, the triggering beats locations were recorded within the Purkinje system.

The important role played by the heart conduction system in the genesis of VF is confirmed by Marrouche et al.[32] They reported on the initiation of VF storm in 29 patients with ischemic cardiomyopathy and remote myocardial infarction. Monomorphic premature ventricular beats trigger VF storm in all patients; they appear to be related to Purkinje-like potentials originating from the scar border zone. Moreover, catheter ablation of these triggering premature beats and/or of potentials in the border zone region, with the aid of the 3-D electroanatomic mapping system, can control and prevent VF storm over a relatively long follow-up.

Histologic abnormalities of the conduction system have been reported in victims of sudden death either with structural disease or with normal heart.[33] The initiating role of the Purkinje system may result from automaticity, re-entry, or triggered activity and is sensitive to various clinical factors such as catecholamines, electrolyte disturbance, drugs, and myocardial ischemia during which Purkinje fibers may survive within necrotic muscle. Purkinje fibers are more resistant to ischemia than myocardial cells, and, when endocardial, may be nourished from cavity blood. Thus, they can remain structurally intact but altered in function, giving rise to triggered activity or afterdepolarization.[34] In the Bansch et al study,[31] a considerable number of radiofrequency pulses were necessary to abolish ventricular premature beats, suggesting that the triggering fibers cover an extensive area at the border of the zone of the infarction and may have different connections to the surrounding myocardial tissue. In animal models, triggered activity from surviving distal Purkinje fiber arborization in the scar border is required to initiate VF.[35]

Ventricular premature beats may also arise from microre-entry caused by coexisting scar and viable myocardium, but the potentials described at ablation sites by all three reports do not resemble potentials in re-entrant circuit, which are usually more fractionated and at much lower frequency.

### Radiofrequency catheter ablation of VT

In the majority of cases of SCD, the cause is the onset of a monomorphic VT which degenerates into VF (Wiggers' stage 1). Thus, preventing the onset of VT by catheter ablation may help to prevent VF episodes and SCD, particularly in patients with ischemic heart disease.

In a recent study, we[36] demonstrated that effective cardiac ablation of tolerated VT in patients with prior myocardial infarction may improve long-term outcome, particularly reducing SCD, even without the ICD device. Hybrid therapy (ablation plus ICD) is therefore necessary when multiple morphology tachycardia was clinically present or induced during ablation.

Furthermore, well-tolerated VT accounts for less than 10% of the total VT population.[37] In recent years, however, the development of new mapping techniques (noncontact mapping, sinus rhythm mapping, electroanatomic mapping) has allowed performance of catheter ablation even in hemodynamically unstable or untolerated VT with different acute and long-term success rate.[38–40]

A particular subgroup is represented by patients with storm of untolerated monomorphic VT. We performed radiofrequency catheter ablation in 17 patients with

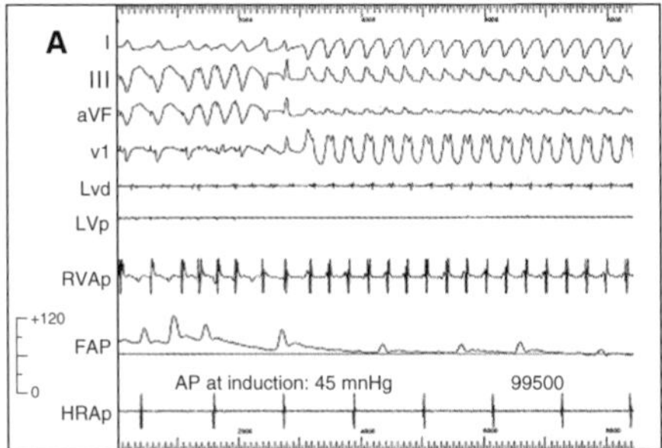


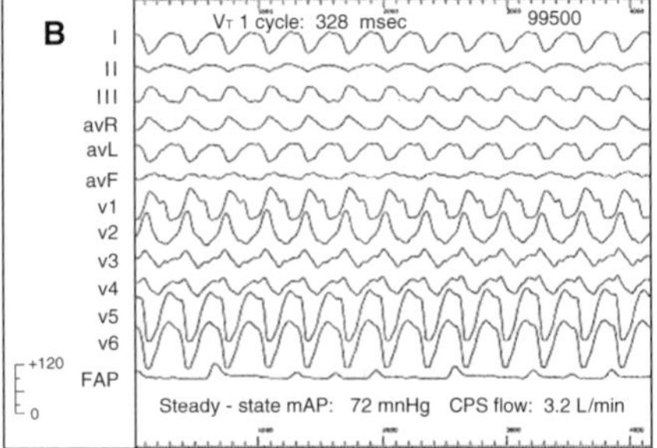


**Figure 3.2** (A) Simultaneous recording of surface ECG, electrograms from left (LV) and right (RVA) ventricle, and from right atrial appendage (HRA), and of arterial blood pressure. Following programmed ventricular stimulation from the right ventricle, while the pCPS was on stand-by, monomorphic ventricular tachycardia was induced and the mean blood pressure dropped to 45 mmHg after few seconds of observation. (B) Simultaneous recording of surface ECG and arterial blood pressure during ventricular tachycardia. The percutaneous CPS was turned on, and the pump speed was gradually increased to provide an average arterial pressure of 70 mmHg.

unstable VT related to ischemic cardiopathy, idiopathic or valvular cardiomyopathy, or right ventricular dysplasia (mean ejection fraction of 35%), using the percutaneous cardiopulmonary support system (pCPS) as hemodynamic support to allow conventional catheter mapping.[41] We demonstrated that pCPS is a safe and efficacious alternative strategy to map and ablate untolerated VT. Furthermore, we observed that during this VT storm, before institution of pCPS, the arterial pressure immediately dropped below 50 mmHg (Figure 3.2). These data suggest that in severely ill patients untolerated monomorphic VT can be sufficient to cause SCD, even in the absence of degeneration to VF (Wiggers' stage 2).

Perhaps decreasing the incidence of VF or VT episodes by catheter ablation may not reduce the need of ICD, but it can decrease the number of therapies delivered and the amount of drugs prescribed, and improve patient quality of life.

## SCD in patients with ICD

It is well known that the ICD improves survival in high-risk cardiac patients. Nevertheless, SCD is still a common mode of death in patients with an ICD.[42] A recent study by Mitchell et al[43] reports that the mode of death in ICD patients is sudden in 28% of cases, and that the most common mechanism is VF or VT treated with an appropriate shock and followed by EMD. It is possible that the postshock EMD is an epiphenomenon arising from some other fatal event, such as large-extent ischemia. However, the authors suggest that many of these deaths result from ICD shocks that are too frequent, too closely spaced or too large in magnitude. This hypothesis is supported by reports of severe hemodynamic deterioration after internal direct-current shocks during ICD implantation, particularly in patients with poor ventricular function.[44] Recognition and prevention of this phenomenon should lead to a reduction in SCD.

## REFERENCES


1. Myerburg RJ, Castellanos A. Cardiac arrest and sudden death. In: Braunwald E, Zipes DP, Libby P, eds. Heart Disease: A Textbook of Cardiovascular Medicine. 6th edn. Philadelphia: WB Saunders, 2001: 890–931.
2. Muller JE, Kaufmann PG, Luepker RV et al., for the Mechanisms Precipitating Acute Cardiac Events participants. Mechanisms precipitating acute cardiac events: review and recommendations of an NHLBI workshop. Circulation 1997; 96: 3233–9.
3. Holmes DR Jr, Davis KB, Mock MB et al. The effect of medical and surgical treatment on subsequent sudden cardiac death in patients with coronary artery disease: a report from the Coronary Artery Surgery Study. Circulation 1986; 73: 1254–63.
4. Theroux P, Fuster V. Acute coronary syndromes: unstable angina and non-Q-wave myocardial infarction. Circulation 1998; 97: 1195–1206.
5. Zipes DP, Wellens HJJ. Sudden cardiac death. Circulation 1998; 98: 2334–51.
6. Chugh SS, Kelly KL, Titus JL. Sudden cardiac death with apparently normal heart. Circulation 2000; 102: 649–54.
7. Stevenson WG, Stevenson LW, Middelkauff HR, Saxon LA. Sudden death prevention in patients with advanced ventricular dysfunction. Circulation 1993; 88: 2953–61.
8. Vassalle M. On the mechanism underlying cardiac standstill: factors determining success or failure of escape pacemakers in the heart. J Am Coll Cardiol 1985; 5(Suppl B): 35.
9. Gettes LS, Cascio WE, Sanders WE. Mechanisms of sudden cardiac death. In: Zipes DP, Jalife J, eds. Cardiac Electrophysiology: From Cell to Bedside. 2nd edn. Philadelphia: WB Saunders, 1995: 527–38.
10. Kothari SS. Electromechanical dissociation. Postgrad Med 1991; 90: 75–8.
11. Josephson M, Wellens HJJ. Implantable defibrillators and sudden cardiac death. Circulation 2004; 109: 2685–91.
12. Myerburg RJ, Kessler KM, Castellanos A. Sudden cardiac death. Structure, function, and time-dependence of risk. Circulation 1992; 85: I2–I10.
13. Zipes DP. Sudden cardiac death. Future approaches. Circulation 1992; 85: I160–I166.
14. Spooner PM, Albert C, Benjamin EJ et al. Sudden cardiac death, genes and arrhythmogenesis: consideration of new population and mechanistic approaches from a National Heart, Lung and Blood Institute workshop. I. Circulation 2001; 103: 2361–4.
15. Spooner PM, Albert C, Benjamin EJ et al. Sudden cardiac death, genes and arrhythmogenesis: consideration of new population and mechanistic approaches from a National Heart, Lung and Blood Institute workshop. II. Circulation 2001; 103: 2447–52.
16. Satoh T, Zipes DP. Unequal atrial stretch in dogs increases dispersion of refractoriness conducive to developing atrial fibrillation. J Cardiovasc Electrophysiol 1996; 7: 833–42.
17. Wiggers CJ, Bell JR, Pine M. Studies of ventricular fibrillation caused by electrical shock. II. Cinematographic and electrocardiographic observation of the natural process in the dog's heart. Its inhibition by potassium and the revival of coordinated beats by calcium. Am J Heart 1930; 5: 351–65.
18. Chen P-S, Wolf PD, Dixon EG et al. Mechanism of ventricular vulnerability to single premature stimuli in open chest dogs. Circ Res 1988; 62: 1191–1209.
19. Lee JJ, Kamjoo K, Hough D et al. Reentrant wave fronts in Wiggers' stage II ventricular fibrillation: characteristics, and mechanism of termination and spontaneous regeneration. Circ Res 1996; 78: 660–75.
20. Worley SJ, Swain JL, Colavita PG et al. Development of an endocardial-epicardial gradient of activation rate during electrically induced sustained ventricular fibrillation in dogs. Am J Cardiol 1985; 55: 813–20.
21. Moe GK. On the multiple wavelet hypothesis of atrial fibrillation. Arch Int Pharmacodyn Ther 1962; 140: 183–8.
22. Choi BR, Nho W, Liu T et al. Life span of ventricular fibrillation frequencies. Circ Res 2002; 91: 339–45.
23. Valderrabano M, Yang J, Omichi C et al. Frequency analysis of ventricular fibrillation in swine ventricles. Circ Res 2002; 90: 213–22.

24. Gray RA, Jalife J, Panfilov AV et al. Mechanisms of cardiac fibrillation. Science 1995; 270: 1222–3.
25. Wu T-J, Lin SW-N, Weiss JN et al. Two types of ventricular fibrillation in isolated rabbit hearts: importance of excitability and action potential duration restitution. Circulation 2002; 106: 1859–66.
26. Chen P-S, Wu T-J, Ting C-T et al. A tale of two fibrillations. Circulation 2003; 108: 2298–303.
27. Grafinkel A, Kim Y-H, Voroshilovsky O et al. Preventing ventricular fibrillation by flattening cardiac restitution. Proc Natl Acad Sci USA 2000; 97: 6061–6.
28. Suddath WO, Deychak Y, Varghese PJ. Electrophysiologic basis by which epinephrine facilitates defibrillation after prolonged episodes of ventricular fibrillation. Ann Emerg Med 2001; 38: 201–6.
29. Haissaguerre M, Shoda M, Jais P et al. Mapping and ablation of idiopathic ventricular fibrillation. Circulation 2002; 106: 962–7.
30. Haissaguerre M, Extramiana F, Hocini M et al. Mapping and ablation of ventricular fibrillation associated with long-QT and Brugada syndromes. Circulation 2003; 108: 925–8.
31. Bansch D, Oyang F, Antz M et al. Successful catheter ablation of electrical storm after myocardial infarction. Circulation 2003; 108: 3011–16.
32. Marrouche NF, Verma A, Wazni O et al. Mode of initiation and ablation of ventricular fibrillation storms in patients with ischemic cardiomyopathy. J Am Coll Cardiol 2004; 43: 1715–20.
33. Moe T. Morgagni–Adams–Stokes attacks caused by transient recurrent ventricular fibrillation in a patient without apparent organic heart disease. Am Heart J 1949; 37: 811–18.
34. Friedman PL, Stewart JR, Wit AL. Spontaneous and induced cardiac arrhythmias in subendocardial Purkinje fibers surviving extensive myocardial infarction in dogs. Circ Res 1973; 33: 612–26.
35. Janse MJ, Kleber AG, Capucci A, Coronel R, Wilms-Schopman F. Electrophysiological basis for arrhythmias caused by acute ischemia. Role of the subendocardium. J Mol Cell Cardiol 1986; 18: 339–55.
36. Della Bella P, De Ponti R, Uriarte JAS et al. Catheter ablation and antiarrhythmic drugs for haemodynamically tolerated post infarction ventricular tachycardia. Long term outcome in relation to acute electrophysiological findings. Eur Heart J 2002; 23: 414–24.
37. Morady F, Harvey M, Kalbfleish SJ et al. Radiofrequency catheter ablation in patients of coronary artery disease. Circulation 1993; 87: 363–72.
38. Della Bella P, Pappalardo A, Riva S et al. Non-contact mapping to guide catheter ablation of untolerated ventricular tachycardia. Eur Heart J 2002; 23: 742–52.
39. Furniss S, Anil Kumar R, Bourke JP et al. Radiofrequency ablation of haemodynamically unstable ventricular tachycardia after myocardial infarction. Heart 2000; 84: 648–52.
40. Marchlinski FE, Callans DJ, Gottlieb CD et al. Linear ablation lesions for control of unmappable ventricular tachycardia in patients with ischemic and nonischemic cardiomyopathy. Circulation 2000; 101: 1288–96.
41. Fassini G, Della Bella P, Trevisi N et al. Long term safety and outcome of hemodynamically-supported catheter ablation for the treatment of untolerated ventricular tachicardia. PACE 2002; 24: 533 (Abstract).
42. Grubman EM, Pavri BB, Shipman T, Britton N, Kocovic DZ. Cardiac death and stored electrograms in patients with third generation implantable cardioverter defibrillators. J Am Coll Cardiol 1998; 32: 1056–62.
43. Mitchell LB, Pineda EA, Titus JL, Bartosch PM, Benditt DG. Sudden death in patients with implantable cardioverter defibrillators. The importance of post shock electromechanical dissociation. J Am Coll Cardiol 2004; 39; 1323–8.
44. Steinbeck G, Dorwarth U, Mattke S et al. Hemodynamic deterioration during ICD implant: predictors of high risk patients. Am Heart J 1994; 127: 1064–7.

# 4

# Is it possible to prevent sudden death? – primary prevention

Kristina Wasmer, Günter Breithardt and Lars Eckardt

Primary prevention of sudden cardiac death (SCD) includes both prevention of cardiac disease and optimal medical therapy once a cardiac disease has been recognized. To discuss all these measures in detail would be beyond the scope of this chapter. Antiarrhythmic drugs and the automated external defibrillator are discussed in separate chapters of this book. This chapter summarizes primarily current knowledge on the implantable cardioverter defibrillator (ICD) for primary prevention of sudden death (Figure 4.1).

## SCD IN PATIENTS WITH STRUCTURAL HEART DISEASE

Most patients who die suddenly have underlying structural heart disease. Coronary artery disease (CAD) and its consequences account for at least 80% of SCD. Other frequent causes are dilated cardiomyopathy, hypertrophic cardiomyopathy, and arrhythmogenic right ventricular dysplasia. SCD may also occur in patients with congenital heart disease, such as tetralogy of Fallot.

### CAD and myocardial infarction

The risk factors for atherosclerotic coronary disease are well known, namely, increasing age, male gender, family history of CAD, increased low-density lipoprotein (LDL) cholesterol, hypertension, smoking and diabetes mellitus. Thus, eliminating these risk factors is part of primary prevention of SCD.

Left ventricular dysfunction is the main risk factor for SCD in patients with CAD. Therefore, limitation of infarct size and prevention of left ventricular dysfunction are the main goals in the treatment of acute myocardial infarction. Thrombolytic treatment in the acute setting of myocardial infarction reduces the risk of future death by 18–50%. The benefit from thrombolytic therapy increases up to 25% when oral aspirin is also administered in the early phase. Successful achievement of vessel patency and TIMI 3 flow results in preservation of left ventricular function, and limitation of scar size, the substrate for late ventricular tachyarrhythmia and SCD.

In post-myocardial infarction studies, *beta-blockers* have been shown to decrease overall mortality and SCD. In a recent analysis[1] of 31 beta-blocker trials, only 13 trials reported data on reduction of SCD. These trials showed a reduction of SCD by 51–43% in patients treated with beta-blockers versus the untreated group.

The use of *angiotensin-converting enzyme inhibitors* (ACE inhibitors) has been investigated in patients with recent myocardial infarction and patients with asymptomatic

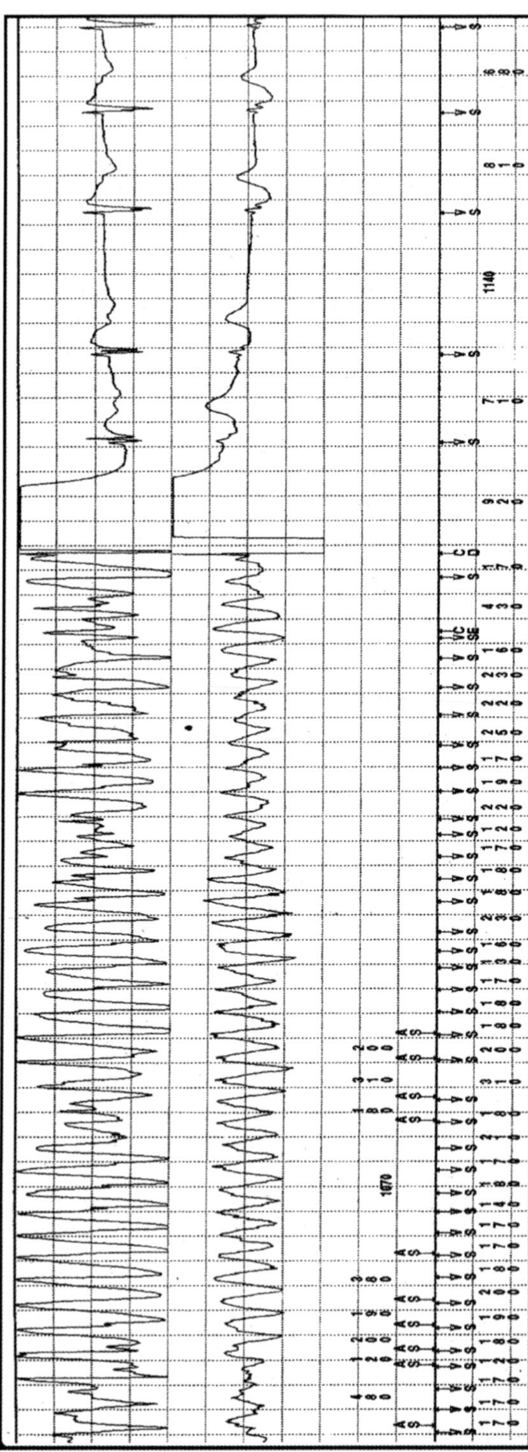

**Figure 4.1** Detection and termination of ventricular fibrillation by an implantable cardioverter defibrillator.

chronic left ventricular dysfunction, as well as in moderate and advanced heart failure. Treatment with ACE inhibitors resulted in a decreased progression to overt heart failure and a decrease in death due to progressive heart failure and SCD. Reduction of SCD by ACE inhibitors was 30–54%, which was statistically significant in some studies.[2,3] The RALES trial[4] showed that spironolactone therapy in patients receiving diuretics, ACE inhibitors and, in most cases, digoxin was associated with a significant reduction in death due to progressive heart failure and SCD.

Three large *statine* trials[5–7] (4S = Scandinavian Simvastatin Survival Study, CARE and LIPID) showed that a reduction of all-cause mortality in patients assigned to treatment with *lipid-lowering agents* was paralleled by a reduction in SCD.

Of the different *antiarrhythmic drugs* that have been evaluated, only beta-blockers and amiodarone have reduced sudden death in myocardial infarction survivors. Class I antiarrhythmic drugs (mexiletine, encainide, flecainide, and moricizine), calcium antagonists, and class III drugs (sotalol and dofetilide) all failed to reduce, or they even increased, the incidence of SCD after myocardial infarction.[8] CAMIAT[9] and EMIAT[10] showed a significant reduction in SCD (35%), but no reduction in overall mortality.

Since its first implantation 25 years ago, the ICD has become the first-choice therapy in patients who survived cardiac arrest. ICD therapy has proven to be superior to antiarrhythmic drugs in mortality reduction in many patient groups.[11,12] Several trials have evaluated the role of prophylactic ICD implantation in post-myocardial infarction patients (Table 4.1).

The first major study was the Multicenter Automatic Defibrillator Implantation Trial (MADIT),[13] which included 196 patients with prior myocardial infarction, left ventricular ejection fraction (LVEF) of ≤35%, nonsustained ventricular tachycardia (VT), and inducible sustained VT upon electrophysiologic study not suppressible by intravenous procainamide. During an average follow-up of 27 months, there were 15 deaths in the ICD group and 39 deaths in the conventional therapy group (the hazard ratio for all-cause mortality associated with the ICD was 0.46). The Coronary Artery Bypass Graft (CABG) Patch Trial[14] randomized 1055 patients with LVEF of ≤35%, no prior VT/ventricular fibrillation, and abnormal signal-averaged ECG scheduled for bypass surgery to either concomitant epicardial ICD implantation or only conventional medical management excluding antiarrhythmic agents. During an average follow-up of 32 ± 16 months, there were 101 deaths in the defibrillator group and 95 in the control group. The hazard ratio for death from any cause was 1.07. There was no benefit from ICD therapy, probably reflecting the important benefit provided by definitive surgical revascularization in reducing myocardial ischemia and improving left ventricular systolic function. MADIT II[15] was designed to evaluate the effect of an implantable defibrillator on survival in patients with prior myocardial infarction and LVEF of ≤30% without requiring documented nonsustained VT or electrophysiologic study. A total of 1232 patients were randomly assigned in a 3:2 ratio to receive either ICD therapy (742 patients) or only conventional medical therapy (490 patients) that included beta-blockers, ACE inhibitors, and lipid-lowering drugs. During an average follow-up of 20 months, the mortality rates were 19.8% in the conventional therapy and 14.2% in the ICD group. The hazard ratio for the risk of death from any cause in the ICD group compared with the conventional-therapy group was 0.69. The effect of ICD therapy was similar in subgroup analyses stratified according to ejection fraction (EF), New York Heart Association (NYHA) functional class and QRS (electrical activation of the ventricle) interval. The Sudden Cardiac Death in Heart Failure Trial

**Table 4.1** Primary prevention trials in patients with coronary artery disease

| Trial | Inclusion criteria | No. of patients | Underlying heart disease | Follow-up (months) | Hazard ratio (risk of death from any cause), 95% confidence interval |
|---|---|---|---|---|---|
| MADIT[13] | EF ≤ 35%, nsVT, EP inducibility, no suppression of induced VT by procainamide | 196 | CAD only | 27 | 0.46<br>0.26–0.82<br>$P = 0.009$ |
| CABG-patch[14] | Elective CABG, positive signal-averaged ECG | 1055 | CAD only | 32 ± 16 | 1.07<br>0.81–1.42<br>$P = 0.64$ |
| MADIT II[15] | EF ≤ 30% | 1232 | CAD only | 20 | 0.69<br>0.51–0.93<br>$P = 0.016$ |
| SCD-HeFT[16] | EF ≤ 35%, NYHA II or III stable heart failure | 2521 | CAD 52% | Median 45.5 | 0.77<br>97.5% confidence interval<br>0.62–0.96<br>$P = 0.007$ |
| DINAMIT[17] | Recent myocardial infarction (6–40 days), EF ≤ 35%, evidence of autonomic imbalance | 674 | CAD only | 30 ± 13 | 1.08<br>0.76–1.55<br>two-sided $P = 0.66$ |
| COMPANION[18] | Class III or IV heart failure, EF ≤ 35%, QRS 120 ms, PR > 150 ms, sinus rhythm, hospitalization for heart failure in the preceding 12 months | 1520 | CAD 59, 54, and 55% | 16 | 0.73<br>0.52–1.04<br>$P = 0.082$<br>ICD vs pharmacologic therapy |
| CARE-HF[19] | EF ≤ 35%<br>NYHA III–IV<br>QRS ≥ 120 ms<br>No atrial arrhythmias | 813 | CAD 36 and 40% | 29.4 | 0.64<br>0.48–0.85<br>$P < 0.002$<br>Medical therapy versus medical therapy plus resynchronization therapy |

(SCD-HeFT)[16] included 2521 patients with left ventricular dysfunction regardless of cause (52% ischemic) and used the presence of heart failure despite medical therapy and a left EF of less than 36% as entry criteria. The median follow-up was 45.5 months. There were 244 deaths (29%) in the placebo group, 240 (28%) in the amiodarone group and 182 (22%) in the ICD group. As compared with placebo, amiodarone was associated with a similar risk of death (hazard ratio of 1.06), and ICD therapy was associated with a decreased risk of death of 23% (hazard ratio of 0.77) and an absolute decrease in mortality reduction of 7.2 percentage points after 5 years in the overall population. The authors noted that the benefit of the ICD in SCD-HeFT appeared to be more marked in patients with less severe congestive heart failure. This finding differs from results of the MADIT II trial, which showed that the benefit of the ICD was greater among patients with class III heart failure.

Although the ICD has been shown to be beneficial in patients with chronic left ventricular dysfunction, this is not the case when the ICD is used very early after myocardial infarction. The DINAMIT trial[17] included 674 patients 6–40 days after myocardial infarction with an EF of 35% or less and impaired cardiac autonomic function and randomized to either ICD therapy or no ICD therapy. During a mean follow-up of 30±13 months, 120 patients died, 62 in the ICD group and 58 in the control group. Prophylactic ICD therapy did not reduce overall mortality (hazard ratio for death of 1.08), although it was associated with a reduction in the rate of death due to arrhythmia (hazard ratio of 0.42).

The addition of a left ventricular lead to provide resynchronization therapy has been shown to improve heart failure and decrease mortality among patients with left ventricular dysfunction and wide QRS complexes. The COMPANION (Comparison of Medical Therapy, Pacing, and Defibrillation in Heart Failure) trial[18] included 1520 patients with nonischemic or ischemic cardiomyopathy, NYHA III–IV, LVEF of ≥35% and QRS of ≥120 ms. They were randomly assigned in a 1:2:2 ratio to receive optimal pharmacologic therapy alone or in combination with cardiac-resynchronization therapy with either a pacemaker or a pacemaker-defibrillator. In the pharmacologic therapy group, 59% of patients had underlying coronary artery disease, 54% in the pacemaker and 56% in the defibrillator group, respectively. For mortality, the median duration of follow-up was 14.8, 16.5 and 16.0 months, respectively. The 1-year mortality rate in the pharmacologic therapy group was 19%. The implantation of a pacemaker was associated with a marginally significant reduction in the risk of death from any cause (hazard ratio of 0.76), whereas the implantation of a pacemaker-defibrillator was associated with a significant 36% reduction in risk (hazard ratio of 0.64). Cardiac resynchronization therapy decreased the combined risk of death from any cause or first hospitalization for heart failure (34% pacemaker group, 40% defibrillator group) and, when combined with ICD, significantly reduced mortality (36% risk reduction of death). In addition, the CARE-HF trial[19] investigated the effect of cardiac resynchronization therapy on morbidity and mortality in patients with left ventricular systolic dysfunction (EF of ≤35%), left ventricular end-diastolic dimension of at least 30 mm, classes III and IV heart failure, and QRS interval of at least 120 ms. A total of 813 patients were included; 36% ($n=144$, medical group) and 40% ($n=165$, medical therapy plus cardiac resynchronization) of patients had heart failure due to ischemic cardiomyopathy. The mortality rate in the medical therapy group was 12.6% at 1 year and 25.1% at 2 years, as compared with 9.7% and 18.0%, respectively, in the cardiac resynchronization group. Calculations based on hazard ratios suggest that, for every nine devices implanted, one death and three hospitalizations for major cardiovascular events are prevented. The benefits were similar among patients with and without ischemic heart disease and in addition to those afforded by pharmacologic therapy.

Based on the results of these ICD trials, the role of prophylactic ICD implantation in primary prevention can be better defined: patients with recent myocardial infarction, as well as patients with poor left ventricular function who require bypass surgery, appear not to benefit from prophylactic ICD implantation. Left ventricular dysfunction is probably reversible in some of these patients, as remodeling of the infarcted myocardium has not yet reached a stable phase or ischemia is treated by bypass surgery. In contrast, patients with a stable substrate (more than 6 months after myocardial infarction) and an EF of less than 31% should be considered for a single-chamber ICD to improve their survival. In patients with advanced heart failure and QRS of ≥120 ms, cardiac resynchronization therapy may reduce mortality. Patients with EF of 31–40% may be further risk stratified by electrophysiologic testing.[20]

## Dilated cardiomyopathy

Patients with dilated cardiomyopathy have a high mortality. In the late 1980s, mortality rates were estimated to be 30% at 1 year.[21] Heart failure therapy with ACE inhibitors, beta-blockers, diuretics and aldosterone antagonists was able to decrease the 1-year mortality to 5–15%.[22] Of these patients, 30–40% die suddenly. Therapeutic strategies for primary prevention of SCD in patients with dilated cardiomyopathy mainly consist of amiodarone and the ICD.

Two studies have evaluated prophylactic ICD implantation in patients with dilated cardiomyopathy. The Cardiomyopathy Trial (CAT)[23] included 104 patients with dilated cardiomyopathy of recent onset (≤9 months) and impaired EF (≤30%) without documented symptomatic ventricular tachyarrhythmia who were randomly assigned to ICD therapy or to a control group. The study revealed that short- and long-term overall mortality rates in patients with dilated cardiomyopathy and significantly impaired left ventricular function were low (long-term survival rate 92%, 86% and 73% in the ICD group and 93%, 80%, and 68% in the control group after 2, 4 and 6 years). ICD therapy did not provide any survival benefit in these patients. AMIOVIRT[24] compared the outcome of 103 patients with dilated cardiomyopathy, EF of ≤35%, asymptomatic nonsustained VT and heart failure NYHA I–III who had been randomized to receive either amiodarone or ICD. Mortality and quality of life were similar in both groups with no statistically significant difference (survival at 1 year 90% vs 96% and at 3 years 88% vs 87% in the amiodarone and ICD groups, respectively) when the trial was aborted after 2 years. The DEFINITE trial[25] randomly assigned 458 patients with dilated cardiomyopathy, EF of ≤36% and premature ventricular complexes or nonsustained VT to standard therapy or standard medical therapy plus a single-chamber ICD. ICD implantation significantly reduced the risk of sudden death from arrhythmia but had no significant reduction in the risk of death from any cause.

The role of prophylactic ICD therapy in patients with heart failure was evaluated in the SCD-HeFT-trial,[16] which was already mentioned. Patients with dilated cardiomyopathy made up 48% of the total patient population ($n = 1191$). Inclusion criteria were NYHA classes II and III heart failure and EF of ≤35%. Patients were randomized to conventional heart failure therapy plus placebo, conventional therapy plus amiodarone, or conventional therapy plus a conservatively programmed, shock-only, single-lead ICD. For the total study population, the ICD significantly decreased the relative risk of death by 23%, resulting in an absolute reduction of 7.2 percentage points at 5 years. The benefit did not vary according to the cause of heart failure. Amiodarone had no beneficial effect on survival. ICD therapy had a significant benefit in patients with NYHA class II, but not in those with NYHA class III heart failure. Cardiac resynchronization therapy with and without the ICD was studied in the COMPANION trial.[18] Details on the study design have been described earlier. About half of the patients in each randomization group had heart failure due to dilated cardiomyopathy. Among these patients, pacemaker-defibrillator therapy was associated with a significantly lower risk of death from any cause than pharmacologic therapy. In the pacemaker group, as compared with the pharmacologic-therapy group, the implantation of a device reduced the risk of death by 9% in the subgroup of patients with dilated cardiomyopathy (as compared to 28% in the coronary artery disease group). Finally, the CARE-HF trial[19] investigated the effect of cardiac-resynchronization therapy on mortality, as mentioned above in the context of post-myocardial infarction patients. Of 813 included patients, 48% in the medical group ($n = 193$) and 43% in the medical therapy plus cardiac resynchronization group ($n = 177$) had heart failure due to dilated cardiomyopathy. Cardiac resynchronization decreased the incidence of sudden death and of death from worsening heart failure, as discussed above. Nevertheless, 7% of patients ($n = 29$) in the resynchronization group died suddenly, so that the authors considered that ICD therapy may have further reduced the risk of sudden death.

An overview of ICD trials in patients with dilated cardiomyopathy is given in Table 4.2. Routine implantation of an ICD cannot be recommended for all patients with dilated cardiomyopathy and reduced EF. Patients with recent onset dilated cardiomyopathy seem to have a good prognosis when treated with medical therapy (CAT)[23] and have no benefit from additional ICD implantation. These patients can be re-evaluated after about 6–9 months with regard to their EF. Asymptomatic patients with left ventricular dysfunction (EF of ≤35%) can be treated with either amiodarone or an implantable defibrillator. Both seem to be equivalent in this patient group. Patients with left ventricular dysfunction and syncope should receive a defibrillator.[26] In patients with dilated cardiomyopathy, left ventricular dysfunction and NYHA II or III heart failure, amiodarone has no favorable effect on survival (SCD-HeFT). These patients should undergo ICD implantation (COMPANION). If indicated, cardiac-resynchronization therapy in addition to the ICD helps to reduce the risk of SCD in patients with dilated cardiomyopathy and moderate or severe heart failure (CARE-HF).

### Hypertrophic cardiomyopathy (HCM)

Hypertrophic cardiomyopathy (HCM) is a relatively common (adult prevalence about 1:500), inherited heart muscle disorder caused by mutations in genes encoding cardiac sacromeric proteins.[27] The natural history of HCM is diverse, but is relatively benign for most patients. SCD is most common in the young (<30 years), and appears to be the most common cause of SCD in young people, including trained competitive athletes.[28] Risk factors for SCD include unexplained syncope related to exertion, especially in children and adolescents with HCM. Extreme wall thickening (maximum dimension of ≥30 mm), abnormal exercise blood pressure response (failure to rise or hypotensive blood pressure) in young patients (<40 years), and nonsustained VT during ambulatory Holter monitoring are markers of increased risk in adults with HCM.[29,30]

**Table 4.2** Primary prevention trials in patients with dilated cardiomyopathy

| Trial | Inclusion criteria | No. of patients | Underlying heart disease | Follow-up (months) | Hazard ratio (risk of death from any cause), 95% confidence interval |
|---|---|---|---|---|---|
| CAT[23] | Symptomatic DCM for ≤9 months, EF ≤30%, no CAD, NYHA class II or III | 104 | DCM only | 23±4 | Not available |
| AMIOVIRT[24] | DCM, EF ≤35%, asymptomatic NSVT, NYHA class I to III | 103 | DCM only | 24±16 | Not available |
| DEFINITE[25] | DCM, EF <36%, history of symptomatic heart failure, NSVT or frequent VES | 458 | DCM only | 29±14 | 0.65<br>0.4–1.06<br>$P=0.08$ |
| SCD-HeFT[16] | EF ≤35%, NYHA II or III stable heart failure | 2521 | DCM 48% | Median 45.5 | 0.77<br>0.62–0.96<br>$P=0.007$ |
| COMPANION[18] | NYHA III or IV heart failure, EF ≤35%, QRS ≥120 ms, PR > 150 ms, sinus rhythm, hospitalization for heart failure in the preceding 12 months | 1520 | DCM 41%, 46%, 45% | 16 | 0.5<br>0.29–0.88<br>$P=0.015$<br>ICD vs pharmacologic therapy |
| CARE-HF[19] | EF ≤35%<br>NYHA III–IV<br>QRS ≥120 ms<br>No atrial arrhythmia | 813 | DCM 48%, 43% | 29.4 | 0.64<br>0.48–0.85<br>$P<0.002$<br>medical therapy vs cardiac resynchronization |

HR=hazard ratio, CAD=coronary artery disease, DCM=dilated cardiomyopathy, NSVT=nonsustained ventricular tachycardia, VES=ventricular extrasystole, NYHA=New York Heart Association classification for heart failure.

Percentage points for the COMPANION trial refer to treatment groups with pharmacologic therapy and resynchronization therapy with a pacemaker and defibrillator, respectively.

Percentage points for the CARE-HF study refer to medical therapy group and medical therapy plus cardiac resynchronization therapy group, respectively.

The ICD is considered the most effective treatment option for the prevention of SCD. It is strongly recommended for patients who survived a prior cardiac arrest. The role of the ICD for primary prevention of SCD is less well defined.[31] A multicenter, retrospective investigation showed a 5% appropriate annual discharge rate in HCM patients implanted for primary prevention (11%/year for secondary prevention), with no sudden deaths.[32] The mean age at initial appropriate shock was only 40 years. The defibrillators remained dormant for prolonged periods before discharging (up to 9 years), emphasizing the unpredictable timing of SCD events in this disease, the potentially long risk period, and the requirement for extended follow-up duration to assess survival in HCM studies. By extrapolation, it has been estimated that within 20 years, at least 40% of the defibrillators implanted prophylactically in young high-risk HCM patients could intervene and abort sudden death.[29]

The Task Force on SCD of the European Society of Cardiology designates the ICD as a class IIa indication for primary prevention of sudden death in high-risk HCM patients.[30] The availability of sufficient data to support a higher classification is unlikely, given that it is impractical to contemplate a prospective, randomized clinical trial of sufficient size to prove definite benefit of the ICD. In the opinion of the ACC/ESC Expert Consensus Committee on HCM,[33] the presence of multiple clinical risk factors justifies aggressive prophylactic treatment with an ICD. In addition, strong consideration for prophylactic ICD is recommended in the presence of one risk factor regarded as major in that patient. Nevertheless, the potential life-saving implications of device implantation in young patients should always be weighed against possible ICD-related complications including the risk of inappropriate shocks and other lead-related problems, as well as the negative psychological impact that can be associated with implants early in life.

### Arrhythmogenic right ventricular cardiomyopathy (ARVC)

Arrhythmogenic right ventricular cardiomyopathy (ARVC) is characterized by regional or global fibro-fatty replacement of the right ventricular myocardium, with or without left ventricular involvement and with relative sparing of the septum.[34] ARVC is one of the major causes of SCD in the age group under 35 years and accounts for approximately 25% of deaths in young athletes. The ECG is characterized by inverted T-waves and a prolonged QRS complex with epsilon waves in the right precordial leads. The disease is manifested in adolescents or young adults with ventricular arrhythmia (Figure 4.2), syncope or cardiac arrest. Strenuous exercise, sport and acute mental stress are major triggering factors of SCD in patients with ARVC. Patients should therefore be strongly discouraged from practicing competitive sports. The primary indication for drug treatment is to alleviate symptoms such as recurrent palpitations. Use of beta-blockers is recommended. Sotalol and amiodarone can be used if beta-blockers prove ineffective. Prospective, randomized studies on antiarrhythmic drug efficacy in ARVC are not available. However, ICD therapy in patients with ARVC has been evaluated in a few small studies, mainly for secondary prevention of SCD. Corrado et al[35] included 132 patients, of whom 10% received a defibrillator after a cardiac arrest, 39% had sustained VT with hemodynamic compromise, and 23% had sustained VT without hemodynamic compromise. Nine percent of patients had nonsustained VT and 3% had a family history of SCD. During follow-up of 39±25 months, 48% of patients received appropriate ICD interventions, which were potentially life-saving in 24% of patients. Interestingly,

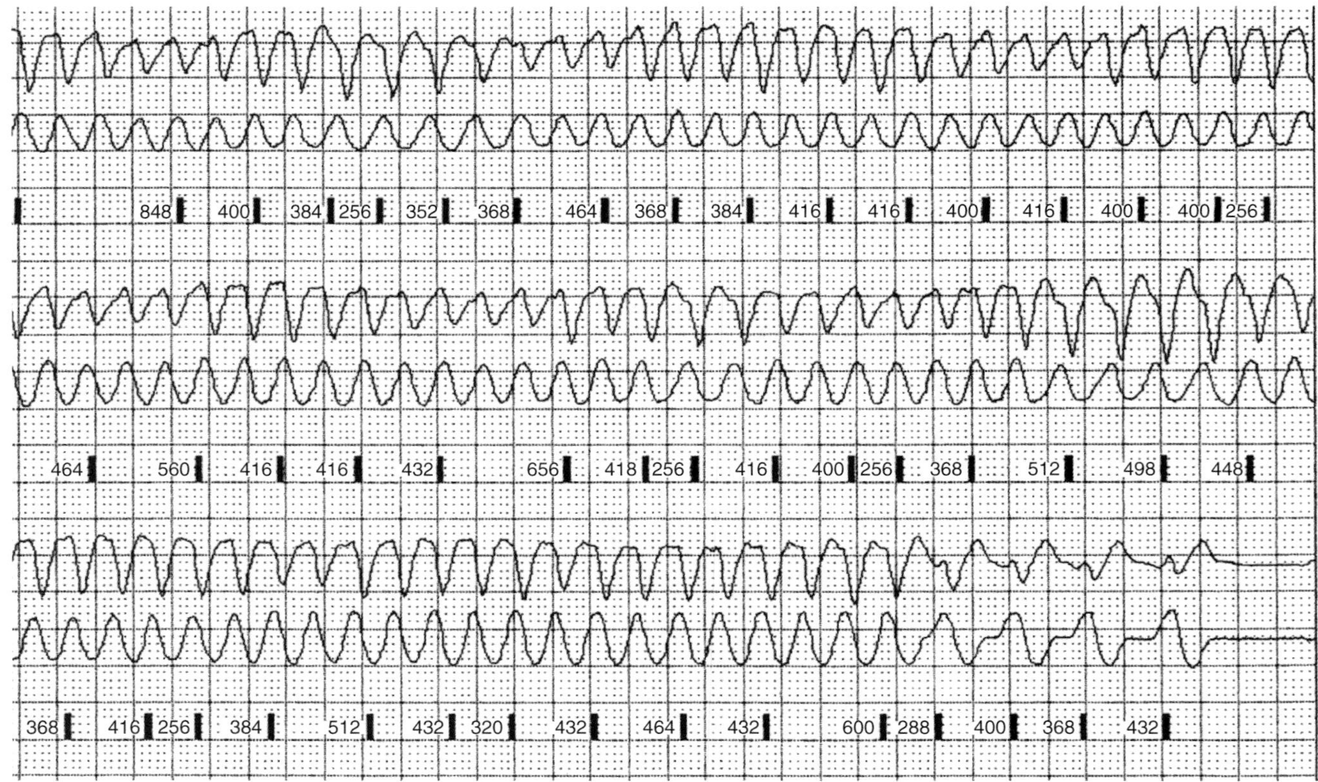


**Figure 4.2** Holter registration of exercise-provoked ventricular tachycardia in a patient with arrhythmogenic right ventricular dysplasia.

ICD intervention rates were similar in patients presenting with cardiac arrest, VT with or without hemodynamic compromise, or unexplained syncope. None of the asymptomatic patients experienced appropriate ICD intervention. Patients with unexplained syncope had an 8% rate of resuscitative ICD intervention. Wichter et al[36] published follow-up data of 60 patients with ARVC who received a defibrillator. The majority of patients had a history of sustained VT or survived cardiac arrest. Only four patients underwent ICD implantation for primary prevention. Two of these four received appropriate ICD therapy during follow-up. Hodgkinson et al[37] investigated the impact of ICD therapy in an autosomal form of familial ARVC. Thirty-five of 48 patients classified as at high risk received a defibrillator in the absence of documented VT. There were no deaths in the ICD group. Male patients were at a significantly higher risk of death than females. Some 47% of the men and 11% of the women had appropriate ICD therapy during follow-up (median time to first discharge was 2.9 years). For male patients, there was no statistical difference in ICD therapy based on whether the ICD was implanted for primary or secondary prevention. The series with the largest subgroup of patients with ARVC who received a prophylactic defibrillator was published by Roguin et al.[38] They evaluated the outcome of 42 patients. In four (10%) patients, ICD was implanted after either resuscitation from cardiac arrest or after an episode of sustained, spontaneous VT, and in 21 (50%) the reason was a syncopal episode. Of the remaining 17 patients (40%), 15 had a history of one or more family sudden deaths, induction of VT during electrophysiologic study and left ventricular involvement. Thirty-three (78%) patients received appropriate ICD therapy during an average 3.5 years of follow-up. There was no difference between secondary and primary prevention indication with regard to appropriate ICD therapy.

The results of these studies suggest that ICD therapy is safe and effective in patients with ARVC not only for secondary prevention but also for primary prevention of sudden death. Potential complications of ICD therapy in patients with ARVC include increased risk of perforation caused by fatty degeneration of the right ventricular wall, difficulty in lead placement owing to inadequate R-wave amplitudes or high pacing thresholds, inadequate sensing or pacing during follow-up, and failure to terminate ventricular arrhythmia owing to rising defibrillation thresholds over time resulting from disease progression. Complication rates of 6–45% have been reported, increasing with longer follow-up periods. Therefore, the indication for ICD implantation in ARVC should weigh the potential benefit against the risk of complications. At this time, the decision to implant an ICD for primary prevention must be based on individual risk assessment, physician judgment, and patient preference.

## SCD IN PATIENTS WITHOUT STRUCTURAL HEART DISEASE

SCD also occurs in patients without overt structural heart disease. Most patients have electrophysiologic abnormalities that can be diagnosed by discrete ECG changes.

### Long-QT syndrome (LQTS)

The long-QT syndrome (LQTS) is characterized by an abnormally prolonged QT interval in the surface ECG, torsade de pointes leading to recurrent syncope and sudden death (Figure 4.3).[39] More than 250 mutations in seven genes (LQTS1–7)

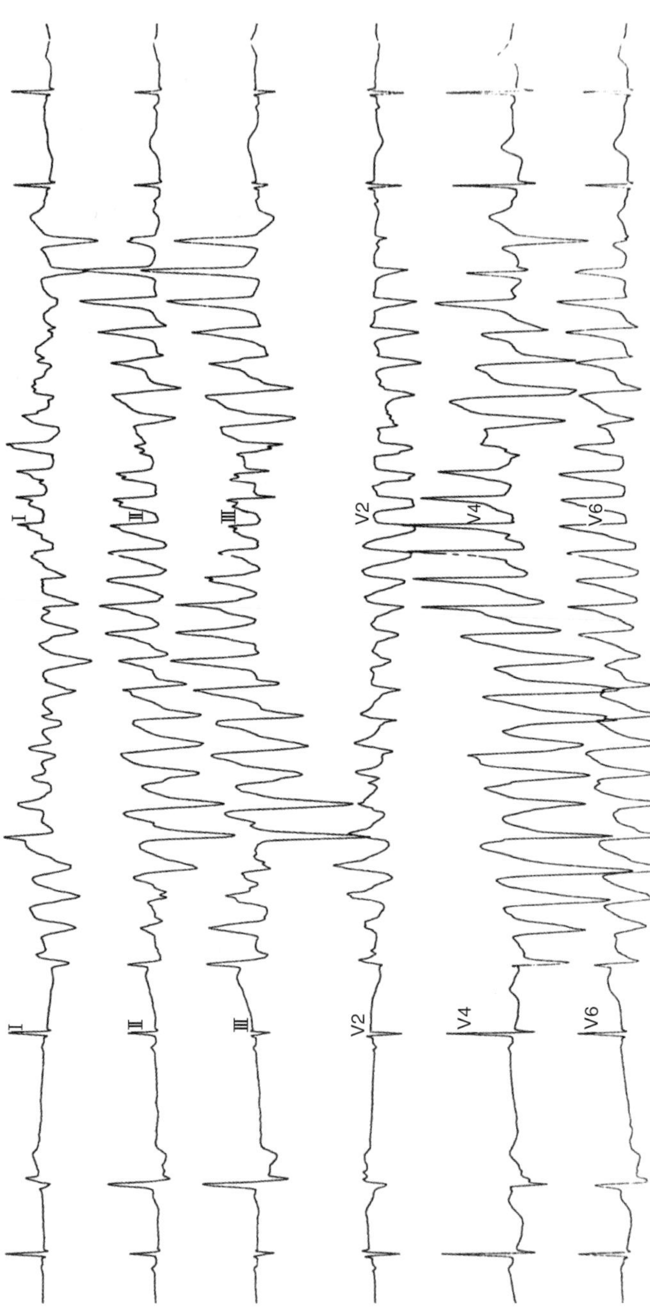


**Figure 4.3** Torsade de pointes ventricular tachycardia in a patient with long-QT syndrome and recurrent syncope.

have been described. Mutations involve genes encoding potassium channels (LQT1, 2, 5 and 6, Jervell Lange-Nielsen (JLN) 1 and 2), sodium channels (LQT3), and ankyrin B (LQT4), which acts as a targeting and anchoring molecule for the sodium channel. Recent genotype–phenotype correlation studies have demonstrated gene-specific triggers for cardiac events.[40] Identification of these triggers may help in suggesting behavioral changes likely to reduce risk. LQT1 patients are at very high risk during exercise, particularly swimming. LQT2 patients are quite sensitive to loud noises, especially when they are asleep or resting. LQT3 appears to be the most malignant variant and the one less effectively managed by beta-blockers.[41] LQT1 and LQT2 have a higher frequency of syncopal events, but their lethality is lower and the protection afforded by beta-blockers, particularly in LQT1, is much higher.

All patients with LQTS – symptomatic, asymptomatic or silent gene carriers – should reduce physical stress, particularly competitive sports. All LQTS patients must avoid the use of drugs that prolong repolarization (listed at websites such as www.longqt.org and www.qtdrugs.org).

Prevention of syncope and sudden death relies on beta-blocker and ICD therapy. A quantification of the actual prevention of SCD by beta-blockers is not available. Retrospective data suggest that mortality 15 years after the first syncope was 9% for the patients treated by antiadrenergic therapy (beta-blockers and/or left cardiac sympathetic denervation) and close to 60% in the group not treated.[42] In another study,[41] mortality data were analyzed in a large group of LQTS patients, including many without symptoms, in whom beta-blockers had been prescribed but who did not necessarily remain on treatment. The 5-year incidence of cardiac arrest or SCD was below 1% for those asymptomatic at treatment initiation, 3% for those who had suffered syncope, and 13% for those who had already had a cardiac arrest. Approximately 25% of the patients who died had been off beta-blockers for a significant amount of time and many of the victims were below 1 year of age. A significant risk of death at first episode strongly suggests the initiation of beta-blocker therapy in asymptomatic patients with clear-cut QT prolongation. No data are available to define the role of prophylactic pharmacologic therapy in asymptomatic gene carriers with normal QT interval.

Prophylactic ICD implantation is considered in patients with syncope despite beta-blocker therapy or in patients with syncope and family history of sudden death. A benefit from ICD therapy has been suggested in retrospective analyses. Zareba et al[43] compared the clinical course of 125 LQTS patients who received a defibrillator because of a prior cardiac arrest ($n=54$), recurrent syncope despite beta-blocker therapy ($n=19$) or other indications (syncope without beta-blockers, SCD in a close family member, $n=52$) with 161 LQTS patients from a registry with similar risk profile (cardiac arrest $n=89$, recurrent syncope despite beta-blocker therapy $n=72$) who did not receive a defibrillator. Data for primary prevention can be taken only from the subgroup with recurrent syncope despite beta-blocker therapy. Mean follow-up was 7 years for patients without ICD and 4 years for patients with ICD. During that time, there were nine deaths in the group without ICD and one in the group with ICD. Among the group with other indications, which consisted of 52 patients with prophylactic ICD implantation, there was one death, which was not related to LQTS. Mönnig et al[44] published a retrospective analysis of 27 LQTS patients who received an ICD. The indication for ICD implantation was a prior cardiac arrest in 17 patients (63%), syncope despite beta-blocker therapy in nine patients (33%), and history of SCD in three close family members in one patient.

**Table 4.3** Recommendations* for primary prevention according to current guidelines (modified from Priori et al[30])

| Cardiac disease | Class I | Class IIa | Class IIb |
|---|---|---|---|
| Post-MI | Beta-blockers, ACE inhibitors, lipid-lowering drugs | Amiodarone | |
| Post-MI+LV dysfunction | Beta-blockers, ACE inhibitors, aldosterone receptor blockers | Amiodarone<br>ICD if EF ≤30% | |
| Post-MI, EF ≤40%, spontaneous NSVT, inducible VT at PES | ICD | | |
| Dilated cardiomyopathy, NSVT | ACE inhibitors, beta-blockers | Aldosterone receptor blockers | Amiodarone, ICD |
| Hypertrophic cardiomyopathy | | ICD | Amiodarone |
| ARVC | | ICD | Antiarrhythmic drugs |
| Long-QT syndrome | Avoid QT-prolonging drugs, sport, beta-blockers | | Pacemaker |
| Brugada syndrome | ICD in patients with syncope/VT | | |

MI=myocardial infarction, ACE inhibitors=angiotensin-converting enzyme inhibitors, NSVT=nonsustained ventricular tachycardia, PES=programmed electrophysiologic stimulation, ICD=implantable cardioverter defibrillator, CHF=congestive heart failure, ARVC=arrhythmogenic right ventricular cardiomyopathy/dysplasia.
*Results of biventricular pacing studies have not yet been incorporated into guidelines.

During a mean follow-up of 65±34 months, there was one death, which was not related to either LQTS or the ICD. The annual ICD discharge rate for patients with a prophylactic ICD was 0.2±0.3 shocks/year compared to 1.3±2.5 shocks/year in those patients who had received the ICD for secondary prevention.

Current guidelines on SCD prevention[30] recommend only beta-blockers for primary prevention of SCD in patients with LQTS; the ICD is reserved only for patients with recurrent syncope despite beta-blocker therapy (Table 4.3).

### Brugada syndrome

Brugada syndrome is characterized by right bundle branch block pattern and ST-segment elevation in leads $V_1$–$V_3$, high risk of SCD in young and otherwise healthy adults, and less risk in infants and children. SCD is caused by rapid polymorphic ventricular arrhythmia mainly occurring at rest or during sleep (Figure 4.4). The syndrome typically manifests itself during adulthood, with a mean age of sudden death of 41±15 years.[45] Brugada syndrome is estimated to be responsible for at least 4% of all sudden deaths and at least 20% of sudden deaths in patients with structurally normal hearts. Data on the natural history and prognosis of patients with the Brugada ECG pattern are controversial,[45–48] probably due to selection bias. Antiarrhythmic agents, such as amiodarone and beta-blockers, have been shown to be ineffective.[49] Class IC antiarrhythmic drugs and class IA agents (probably with

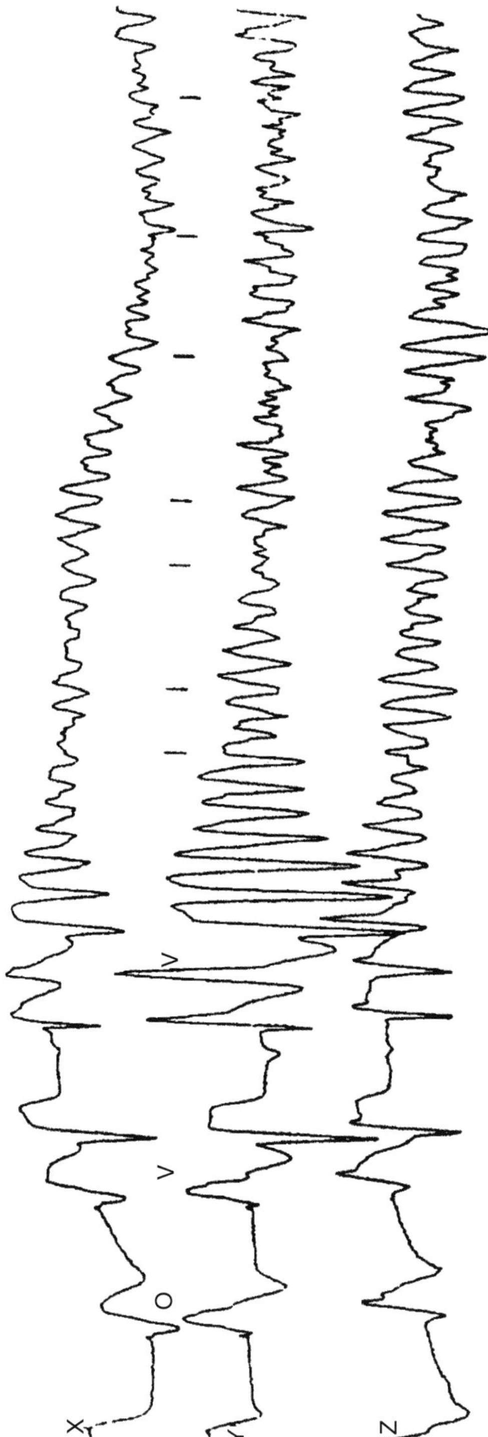


**Figure 4.4** Polymorphic ventricular tachycardia in a patient with Brugada syndrome.

the exception of quinidine) are contraindicated. Currently, the ICD is the only proven effective treatment for the disease. Current recommendations for primary prevention are summarized in a report on a consensus conference.[49] Patients with spontaneous history of syncope, seizure or nocturnal agonal respiration should receive an ICD after noncardiac causes of these symptoms have been ruled out. Controversy exists on whether asymptomatic patients should receive an ICD. According to recommendations made by the Brugada group,[45,46] asymptomatic patients displaying a Brugada ECG (either spontaneously or after sodium channel blockade) should receive an ICD based on inducibility during an electrophysiologic study. Recent follow-up studies of two other groups[47,48] found a relatively low rate of cardiac events in asymptomatic patients (0.8%). Both groups concluded from their data that the electrophysiologic study is not helpful in identifying patients at risk of SCD. They recommend that asymptomatic patients be closely followed up. Long-term follow-up of patient data collected in different registries must be awaited before definite recommendations can be made.

### Other cardiac entities associated with SCD

In addition to the cardiac abnormalities discussed above, SCD may occur in patients without structural heart disease (e.g., idiopathic ventricular fibrillation, catecholaminergic polymorphic VT), those with congenital heart disease (with and without surgical correction) and those with electrophysiologic abnormalities (e.g., Wolff-Parkinson-White (WPW) syndrome, short-QT syndrome). Data are sparse in these patients. Patients with idiopathic ventricular fibrillation cannot be identified in advance, rendering primary prevention impossible. Patients with catecholaminergic polymorphic VT have a high SCD risk despite beta-blocker therapy and should receive a defibrillator once they have been identified.[50] Primary prevention recommendations cannot be made because patient groups are too small or cannot be recognized, as in the case of idiopathic ventricular fibrillation.

## SUMMARY AND CONCLUSION

Is it possible to prevent SCD? – With the introduction of the ICD, we have a device with almost 100% efficacy to prevent death from arrhythmia. The main problem with primary prevention, though, is the identification of the patient who will benefit from the device. The role of prophylactic defibrillator implantation is best defined for patients with coronary artery disease after myocardial infarction. Many sudden deaths can be prevented in this patient group. Still, none of the risk-stratifying criteria can identify all patients at risk, and many ICDs will be implanted that will never be used. For all other patient groups, the role of prophylactic ICD implantation is less well defined. Patients with idiopathic ventricular fibrillation cannot be identified in advance, and many patients with Brugada syndrome, long-QT syndrome and hypertrophic cardiomyopathy may not be identified because they are asymptomatic prior to an arrhythmic event or just not recognized by a primary physician. In addition, not all sudden deaths are due to tachyarrhythmia. Bradyarrhythmia is thought to account for up to 20% of documented SCD.[51]

In summary, many sudden deaths can be prevented by following current guidelines. But primary prevention continues to be difficult. Patient registries and further trials will help to clarify the role of the ICD in primary prevention of SCD.

## REFERENCES

1. Freemantle N, Cleland JG, Young P et al. Beta-blockade after myocardial infarction: systematic review and meta-regression analysis. BMJ 2001; 318: 1730–7.
2. Ambrosioni E, Borghi C, Magnani B. The effect of the angiotensin-converting-enzyme inhibitor zofenopril on mortality and morbidity after anterior myocardial infarction. The Survival in Myocardial Infarction (SMILE) Study Investigators. N Engl J Med 1995; 332: 80–5.
3. Kober L, Torp-Pedersen C, Carlsen JE et al. A clinical trial of the angiotensin-converting-enzyme inhibitor trandolapril in patients with left ventricular dysfunction after myocardial infarction. Trandolapril Cardiac Evaluation (TRACE) Study Group. N Engl J Med 1995; 333: 1670–7.
4. Pitt B, Zannad F, Remme WJ. The effect of spironolactone on morbidity and mortality in patients with severe heart failure. Randomized Aldactone Evaluation Study Investigators. N Engl J Med 1999; 341: 709–17.
5. Randomised trial of cholesterol lowering in 4444 patients with coronary heart disease: the Scandinavian Simvastatin Survival Study (4S). Lancet 1994; 344: 1383–9.
6. Sacks FM, Pfeffer MA, Moye LA et al. The effect of pravastatin on coronary events after myocardial infarction in patients with average cholesterol levels. Cholesterol and Recurrent Events Trial investigators. N Engl J Med 1996; 335: 1001–9.
7. Prevention of cardiovascular events and death with pravastatin in patients with coronary heart disease and a broad range of initial cholesterol levels. The Long-Term Intervention with Pravastatin in Ischemic Disease (LIPID) Study Group. N Engl J Med 1998; 339: 1349–57.
8. Echt DS, Liebson PR, Mitchell LB et al. Mortality and morbidity in patients receiving encainide, flecainide, or placebo. The Cardiac Arrhythmia Suppression Trial. N Engl J Med 1991; 324: 781–8.
9. Cairns JA, Connolly SJ, Roberts R et al. Randomised trial of outcome after myocardial infarction in patients with frequent or repetitive ventricular premature depolarisations: CAMIAT. Canadian Amiodarone Myocardial Infarction Arrhythmia Trial Investigators. Lancet 1997; 349: 675–82.
10. Julian DG, Camm AJ, Frangin J et al. Randomized trial of effect of amiodarone on mortality in patients with left ventricular dysfunction after recent myocardial infarction: EMIAT. Lancet 1997; 349: 667–74.
11. The Antiarrhythmic Versus Implantable Defibrillator (AVID) investigators. A comparison of antiarrhythmic drug therapy with implantable cardioverter defibrillators in patients resuscitated from near-fatal ventricular arrhythmias. N Engl J Med 1997; 337: 1576–83.
12. Kuck KH, Cappato R, Siebels J, Rüppel R, for the CASH investigators. Randomized comparison of antiarrhythmic drug therapy with implantable defibrillators in patients resuscitated from cardiac arrest. Circulation 2000; 102: 748–54.
13. Moss AJ, Hall WJ, Cannom DS et al. Improved survival with an implanted defibrillator in patients with coronary artery disease at high risk for ventricular arrhythmia. Multicenter Automatic
Defibrillator Implantation Trial Investigators. N Engl J Med 1996; 335(26): 1933–40.
14. Bigger JT. Prophylactic use of implanted cardiac defibrillators in patients at high risk for ventricular arrhythmias after coronary-artery bypass graft surgery. Coronary Artery Bypass Graft (CABG) Patch Trial Investigators. N Engl J Med 1997; 337: 1569–75.
15. Moss AJ, Zareba W, Hall WJ et al. Multicenter Automatic Defibrillator Implantation Trial II Investigators. Prophylactic implantation of a defibrillator in patients with myocardial infarction and reduced ejection fraction. N Engl J Med 2002; 346(12): 877–83.
16. Bardy GH, Lee KL, Mark DB et al. Amiodarone or an implantable cardioverter-defibrillator for congestive heart failure. N Engl J Med 2005; 352(3): 225–37.
17. Hohnloser SH, Kuck KH, Dorian P et al. Prophylactic use of an implantable cardioverter-defibrillator after acute myocardial infarction (DINAMIT). N Engl J Med 2004; 351(24): 2481–8.

18. Bristow MR, Saxon LA, Boehmer J et al. Cardiac-resynchronization therapy with or without an implantable defibrillator in advanced chronic heart failure. N Engl J Med 2004; 350(21): 2140–50.
19. Cleland JGF, Daubert JC, Erdmann E et al for the Cardiac Resynchronization – Heart Failure (CARE-HF) Study Investigators. The effect of cardiac resynchronization on morbidity and mortality in heart failure. N Engl J Med 2005; 352(15): 1539–49.
20. Buxton AE, Lee KL, Fisher JD et al. A randomized study of the prevention of sudden death in patients with coronary artery disease. Multicenter Unsustained Tachycardia Trial Investigators. N Engl J Med 1999; 341: 1882–90.
21. Fazio G, Veltri EP, Tomaselli G et al. Long-term follow-up of patients with nonischemic dilated cardiomyopathy and ventricular tachyarrhythmias treated with implantable cardioverter defibrillators. PACE 1991; 14: 1905–10.
22. Dec GW, Fuster V. Idiopathic dilated cardiomyopathy. N Engl J Med 1994; 331(23): 1564–75.
23. Bänsch D, Antz M, Boczor S et al. Primary prevention of sudden cardiac death in idiopathic dilated cardiomyopathy: the cardiomyopathy trial (CAT). Circulation 2002; 105: 1453–8.
24. Strickberger SA, Hummel JD, Bartlett TG et al. Amiodarone versus implantable cardioverter-defibrillator: randomized trial in patients with nonischemic dilated cardiomyopathy and asymptomatic nonsustained ventricular tachycardia – AMIOVERT. J Am Coll Cardiol 2003; 41: 1707–12.
25. Kadish A, Dyer A, Daubert J et al. for the Defibrillators in Non-Ischemic Cardiomyopathy Treatment Evaluation (DEFINITE) Investigators. Prophylactic defibrillator implantation in patients with nonischemic dilated cardiomyopathy. N Engl J Med 2004; 350(21): 2151–8.
26. Knight BP, Goyal R, Pelosi F et al. Outcome of patients with nonischemic dilated cardiomyopathy and unexplained syncope treated with an implantable cardioverter defibrillator. J Am Coll Cardiol 1999; 33: 1964–70.
27. Spirito P, Seidman CE, McKenna et al. The management of hypertrophic cardiomyopathy. N Engl J Med 1997; 336: 775–85.
28. Maron BJ, Shirani J, Poliac LC et al. Sudden death in young competitive athletes: clinical, demographic and pathological profiles. JAMA 1996; 276: 199–204.
29. Spirito P, Bellone P, Harris KM et al. Magnitude of left ventricular hypertrophy predicts the risk of sudden cardiac death in hypertrophic cardiomyopathy. N Engl J Med 2000; 324: 1778–85.
30. Priori SG, Aliot E, Blomstrom-Lundqvist C et al. Task force on sudden cardiac death of the European Society of Cardiology. Eur Heart J 2001; 22: 1374–1450.
31. Maron BJ, Estes NAM III, Maron MS et al. Primary prevention of sudden death as a novel treatment strategy in hypertrophic cardiomyopathy. Circulation 2003; 107: 2872–5.
32. Maron BJ, Shen WK, Link MS et al. Efficacy of implantable cardioverter-defibrillators for the prevention of sudden death in patients with hypertrophic cardiomyopathy. N Engl J Med 2000; 342: 365–73.
33. Maron BJ, McKenna WJ, Danielson GK et al. ACC/ESC clinical expert consensus document on hypertrophic cardiomyopathy: a report of the American College of Cardiology Task Force on Clinical Expert Consensus Documents and the European Society of Cardiology Committee for Practice Guidelines (Committee to Develop an Expert Consensus Document on Hypertrophic Cardiomyopathy). J Am Coll Cardiol 2003; 42(9): 1965–91.
34. McKenna WJ, Thiene G, Nava A et al. Diagnosis of arrhythmogenic right ventricular dysplasia/cardiomyopathy. Task Force of the Working Group on Myocardial and Perimyocardial Disease of the European Society of Cardiology and the Scientific Council on Cardiomyopathies of the International Society and Federation of Cardiology. Br Heart J 1994; 71: 215–8.
35. Corrado D, Loira L, Link MS et al. Implantable cardioverter-defibrillator therapy for prevention of sudden death in patients with arrhythmogenic right ventricular cardiomyopathy/dysplasia. Circulation 2003; 108: 3084–91.

36. Wichter T, Paul M, Wollmann C et al. Implantable cardioverter/defibrillator therapy in arrhythmogenic right ventricular cardiomyopathy. Single-center experience of long-term follow-up and complications in 60 patients. Circulation 2004; 109: 1503–8.
37. Hodgkinson KA, Parfrey PS, Bassett AS et al. The impact of implantable cardioverter-defibrillator therapy on survival in autosomal-dominant arrhythmogenic right ventricular cardiomyopathy (ARVD5). J Am Coll Cardiol 2005; 45: 400–8.
38. Roguin A, Bomma CS, Nasir K et al. Implantable cardioverter-defibrillators in patients with arrhythmogenic right ventricular dysplasia/cardiomyopathy. J Am Coll Cardiol 2004; 43: 1843–52.
39. Camm AJ, Janse MJ, Roden DM et al. Congenital and acquired long QT syndrome. Eur Heart J 2000; 21: 1232–7.
40. Schwartz PJ, Priori SG, Spazzolini C et al. Genotype–phenotype correlation in the long-QT syndrome: gene-specific triggers for life-threatening arrhythmias. Circulation 2001; 103: 89–95.
41. Moss AJ, Zareba W, Hall WJ et al. Effectiveness and limitations of beta-blocker therapy in congenital long-QT syndrome. Circulation 2000; 101: 616–23.
42. Schwartz PJ. Idiopathic long QT syndrome: progress and questions. Am Heart J 1985; 109: 399–411.
43. Zareba W, Moss AJ, Daubert JP et al. Implantable cardioverter defibrillator in high-risk long QT syndrome patients. J Cardiovasc Electrophysiol 2003; 14: 337–41.
44. Mönnig G, Köbe J, Löher A et al. Implantable cardioverter-defibrillator therapy in patients with congenital long-QT syndrome: a long-term follow-up. Heart Rhythm 2005; 2: 497–504.
45. Brugada J, Brugada R, Antzelevitch C et al. Long-term follow-up of individuals with the electrocardiographic pattern of right bundle branch block and ST-segment elevation in precordial leads V1–V3. Circulation 2002; 105: 73–8.
46. Brugada J, Brugada R, Brugada P. Determinants of sudden cardiac death in individuals with the electrocardiographic pattern of Brugada syndrome and no previous cardiac arrest. Circulation 2003; 108: 3092–6.
47. Priori SG, Napolitano C, Gasparini M et al. Natural history of Brugada syndrome: insights for risk stratification and management. Circulation 2002; 105: 1342–7.
48. Eckardt L, Probst V, Smits JPP et al. Long-term prognosis of individuals with right precordial ST segment-elevation Brugada syndrome. Circulation 2005; 111: 257–63.
49. Antzelevitch C, Brugada P, Borggrefe M et al. Brugada syndrome. Report on the second consensus conference. Circulation 2005; 111: 659–70.
50. Francis J, Sancar V, Nair VK et al. Catecholaminergic polymorphic ventricular tachycardia. Heart Rhythm 2005; 2: 550–4.
51. Bayes DL, Coumel P, Leclercq JF. Ambulatory sudden cardiac death: mechanisms of production of fatal arrhythmia on the basis of data from 157 cases. Am Heart J 1989; 117: 151–9.

# 5

# The pharmacologic approach to patients at risk of sudden cardiac death: not only antiarrhythmic drugs

Giuseppe Boriani, Cinzia Valzania, Mauro Biffi, Cristian Martignani, Igor Diemberger, Matteo Bertini, Matteo Ziacchi, Giulia Domenichini, Claudio Rapezzi and Angelo Branzi

## INTRODUCTION

Sudden cardiac death (SCD) is the most common cause of death in developed western countries.[1,2] More than 3 million people are thought to die from SCD each year, worldwide, with a survival rate lower than 1%.[2] Whereas a drop was recorded in total cardiac mortality in the USA between 1989 and 1999, the proportion of deaths with the characteristics of SCD increased by up to 47%.[3]

Improved knowledge of the epidemiology of SCD has been the object of a series of studies,[1,2] which were able to identify high-risk groups of subjects (i.e., subsets of patients with higher incidence of SCD). As reported in detail by Myerburg et al,[1] groups of subjects who definitely have a relevant risk of SCD include patients with previous myocardial infarctions associated with left ventricular (LV) dysfunction and other high-risk markers; patients with a recent ventricular tachyarrhythmia or recent cardiac arrest; and patients with LV dysfunction or heart failure. However, in absolute terms, population subgroups with lower fatality rates account for the largest numbers of SCD victims each year.[1] Consequently, highly selective interventions such as implantable cardioverter defibrillators, whose efficacy has been supported by scientific evidence,[2] have the inherent limitation of targeting only a relatively small proportion of the subjects expected to develop SCD. Despite current efforts to find more sensitive and specific markers of risk in the overall population, the epidemiologic profile of SCD constitutes a major obstacle to any attempt to reduce the overall burden of this form of mortality, especially in the less compromised subsets of patients. Since cardioverter-defibrillators may be considered only in relatively selected patients, medical treatments need to be identified to reduce the burden of SCD in a broader population. Antiarrhythmic agents have failed to improve overall survival through a reduction of SCD, and even amiodarone has recently shown its limitations.[4]

Within this complex scenario, there is growing interest in a series of medications bearing non-antiarrhythmic indications that could indirectly have a positive impact on SCD. Although most of these agents do not have direct, marked electrophysiologic effects on the myocardial fibers, complex interactions exist between substrate, triggers and modulating factors involved in the pathophysiology of SCD. This is an important issue guiding the current interest in this field.

## BETA-BLOCKERS

The cardiovascular benefits of beta-blockers are related to their selective binding to β-adrenoceptors, producing a competitive and reversible antagonism of the effects of β-adrenergic stimulation in various tissues.[5] Thus, the prevention of the cardiotoxic effects of catecholamines plays a central role in the antiarrhythmic action of these drugs. Beta-blockers exert an antiischemic action by reducing heart rate, cardiac contractility and systolic blood pressure. In addition, they induce a reduction of renin release and angiotensin II and aldosterone production by blocking the β1-adrenoceptors on renal juxtaglomerular cells. The improvement in LV structure and function, by decreasing ventricular size and increasing ejection fraction, also plays an important role in the prevention of arrhythmic events. Thus, the antiarrhythmic effects of beta-blockers are mainly related to direct cardiac electrophysiologic effects (reduced heart rate, decreased spontaneous firing of ectopic pacemakers, slowed conduction and increased refractory period of the atrioventricular node), in addition to a reduction of sympathetic drive and myocardial ischemia.[5] Several trials have shown that beta-blockers reduce the risk of hospitalization and death in heart-failure patients. The effects of beta-blocker therapy on all-cause mortality and SCD are summarized in Table 5.1.

While the CIBIS trial[6] showed a nonsignificant trend toward lower mortality in the bisoprolol group, the CIBIS II trial,[7] which enrolled a larger number of patients, showed that treatment with bisoprolol is associated with a significant reduction in all-cause mortality and SCD in patients with heart-failure symptoms and ejection fraction of 35% or less. In this trial, treatment effects were independent of the severity of heart failure etiology. In the MERIT-HF trial,[8] metoprolol, prescribed in addition to standard therapy, significantly reduced both all-cause mortality and SCD in patients with NYHA functional class II–IV symptoms and ejection fraction of 40% or less.

The previously reported benefits of beta-blockers with regard to morbidity and mortality in patients with mild-to-moderate heart failure have been confirmed also in patients with severe heart failure. In the COPERNICUS trial,[9] carvedilol significantly reduced all-cause mortality in patients with NYHA functional class IV symptoms and ejection fraction of 25% or less. The BEST trial[10] evaluated the effects of bucindolol in patients with moderate-to-severe heart failure and low ejection fraction; the study was terminated early in accordance with the recommendations of the safety-monitoring board, influenced by information accruing from other studies of beta-blockers in chronic heart failure. At the time of this recommendation, there was no significant difference in mortality between patients treated with bucindolol or placebo.

The CAPRICORN trial[11] showed a reduction in all-cause and cardiovascular mortality in patients undergoing long-term treatment with carvedilol in addition to standard therapy after acute myocardial infarction complicated by LV systolic dysfunction. Recently, in the COMET trial,[12] in patients with chronic heart failure, carvedilol showed a significantly greater beneficial effect on survival than metoprolol.

**Table 5.1** Main prospective trials of beta-blockers in prevention of mortality and SCD

| Acronym/title | No. patients | Follow-up | Endpoint | *P* | RRR (95% CI) |
|---|---|---|---|---|---|
| CIBIS/Cardiac Insufficiency Bisoprolol Study (1994) | 641 | 1.9 years | All-cause death<br>SCD | 0.22<br>N.S. | 21% (−8% to 49%)<br>11% (−52% to 75%) |
| CIBIS II/Cardiac Insufficiency Bisoprolol Study II (1999) | 2647 | 1.3 years | All-cause death<br>SCD | <0.0001<br>0.0011 | 32% (16% to 47%)<br>43% (17% to 69%) |
| MERIT-HF/Metoprolol CR/XL Randomized Intervention Trial in Congestive Heart Failure (1999) | 3991 | 1 year | All-cause death<br>SCD | 0.00009<br>0.0002 | 32% (16% to 49%)<br>39% (18% to 60%) |
| BEST/Beta-Blocker Evaluation of Survival Trial Investigators (2001) | 2708 | 2.0 years | All-cause death<br>SCD | 0.10<br>0.21 | 8% (−2% to 19%)<br>11% (−7% to 28%) |
| CAPRICORN/ Carvedilol Post-Infarct Survival Control in Left Ventricular Dysfunction (2001) | 1959 | 1.3 years | All-cause death<br>SCD | 0.031<br>0.098 | 22% (2% to 42%)<br>26% (−5% to 56%) |
| COPERNICUS/ Carvedilol Prospective Randomized Cumulative Survival Study (2001) | 2289 | 10.4 months | All-cause death | 0.0014 | 33% (16% to 50%) |
| COMET/Carvedilol or Metoprolol European Trial (2003) | 1511 | 58 months | All-cause death | 0.002 | 14% (6% to 23%) |

CI = confidence interval; N.S. = not significant; RRR = relative risk reduction; SCD = sudden cardiac death

Several meta-analyses[13–18] showed that beta-blocker therapy is associated with clinically meaningful reductions in mortality and morbidity in patients with congestive heart failure. In a meta-analysis[13] of 18 double-blind, placebo-controlled, parallel-group trials of beta-blockers in heart failure, treatment with beta-blockers provided a 32% reduction in the risk of death and a 37% reduction in the combined risk of death or hospitalization for heart failure. A further meta-analysis of 31 beta-blocker trials[17] showed that only 13 trials reported data on SCD reduction, with a reduction from 51% to 43% in patients treated with beta-blockers versus the untreated group.

Since the beneficial effects of beta-blockers have been established beyond any doubt by several randomized, controlled trials, the ESC guidelines[19] recommend

**Table 5.2** Main prospective trials of aldosterone antagonists in prevention of mortality and SCD

| Acronym/title | No. patients | Follow-up | Endpoint | *P* | RRR (95% CI) |
|---|---|---|---|---|---|
| RALES/Randomized Aldactone Evaluation Study Investigators (1999) | 1663 | 1 year | SCD | 0.02 | 20% (2% to 38%) |
| | | | Death from CHD | <0.001 | 11% (4% to 18%) |
| | | | All-cause death | <0.001 | 16% (6% to 27%) |
| EPHESUS/Eplerenone post-Acute Myocardial Infarction Heart Failure Efficacy and Survival Study (2003) | 6642 | 16 months | SCD | 0.03 | 24% (0 to 47%) |
| | | | Death from CHD | 0.005 | 26% (14% to 38%) |
| | | | All-cause death | 0.008 | 25% (15% to 35%) |

CHD = coronary heart disease; CI = confidence interval; RRR = relative risk reduction; SCD = sudden cardiac death

beta-blockers (class I) for primary/secondary prevention of SCD in patients with previous myocardial infarction with or without LV dysfunction.

## ALDOSTERONE ANTAGONISTS

At least three mechanisms exist whereby aldosterone antagonists can bring about a reduction of SCD.[20] Most importantly, these drugs exert sympatholytic effects by increasing cardiac norepinephrine uptake and inactivation. Additionally, aldosterone antagonists reduce both vascular and cardiac fibrosis, and help prevent angiotensin II-induced microangiopathic injury. In fact, spironolactone decreases circulating levels of procollagen type III N-terminal amino peptide (PIIINP), a marker of vascular collagen turnover.[21] Aldosterone antagonists could also provide benefit by alleviating vascular endothelial dysfunction, as aldosterone is thought to reduce nitric oxide production.[22]

The effects of aldosterone antagonists on SCD have been assessed in two randomized, placebo-controlled trials. The RALES trial evaluated the effects of spironolactone in patients with congestive heart failure,[23] while EPHESUS focused on the use of eplerenone in myocardial infarction survivors with LV dysfunction.[24] Both interventions led to valuable reductions in both all-cause mortality and death from SCD. In Table 5.2, the effects of these two interventions on three different measures of survival (all-cause mortality, SCD, and death from congestive heart failure) have been again expressed in terms of reductions in relative and absolute risk, and number needed to treat. Based on the results of these trials, the ESC guidelines[19] recommend aldosterone antagonists (class I) for primary prevention of SCD in patients with previous myocardial infarction and LV dysfunction.

## ANGIOTENSIN-CONVERTING ENZYME (ACE) INHIBITORS

The antiarrhythmic effects of ACE inhibitors also seem to be mediated by several mechanisms.[20] These drugs exert a sympatholytic effect by reducing the level of circulating norepinephrine as well as angiotensin II, which facilitates adrenergic neurotransmission. Baroreflex sensitivity is increased by ACE inhibitors, thereby reducing sympathetic tone, and enhancing vagal tone. Further benefits may derive from the direct electrophysiologic effects of ACE inhibitors (reduction of iK current, enhancement of L-type calcium current). Some of the beneficial effects associated with ACE inhibitor treatment may be related to protection against the potassium depletion brought about by diuretics. ACE inhibitors also help reduce LV volumes and fibrosis during the remodeling process following myocardial infarction.

A large series of clinical trials have uniformly shown that ACE inhibitors provide survival benefits in patients with congestive heart failure or myocardial infarction. In Table 5.3, the trial results are again expressed in terms of reductions in relative and absolute risks (of various endpoints), and the numbers needed to treat.

Regarding congestive heart failure, in the placebo-controlled CONSENSUS trial[25] enalapril reduced overall mortality in patients with NYHA class IV, but no difference was seen in the incidence of SCD. In the SOLVD trial[26] administration of enalapril also reduced the overall mortality of patients in NYHA II–III. The largest reduction regarded deaths attributed to progressive heart failure (no significant difference was detected in deaths from arrhythmia without worsening heart failure). In a separate study by the SOLVD group regarding patients with asymptomatic LV dysfunction,[27] significant benefits from enalapril administration could be found only in terms of progression to symptomatic heart failure and need for hospitalization, while cardiovascular mortality appeared to be unaffected. The V–HeFT II study[28] compared enalapril with an isosorbide/hydralazine combination: the lower overall mortality in the enalapril arm was mainly attributable to a reduction in SCD (this study should be interpreted with caution because of the absence of a placebo arm). In the setting of myocardial infarction, the placebo-controlled SAVE trial[29] showed that captopril can reduce overall mortality in patients with LV dysfunction without overt heart failure or symptoms of myocardial ischemia. Analogous benefits in patients with clinical evidence of heart failure at any time after an acute myocardial infarction were recorded in the AIRE[30] and TRACE[31] trials (after administration of ramipril or trandolapril). GISSI-3,[32] ISIS-4,[33] and SMILE trial[34] showed positive effects of ACE inhibitors on mortality in broader populations of myocardial infarction patients with or without LV dysfunction.

In a meta-analysis[35] of 15 randomized, controlled trials comparing ACE inhibitors with placebo in patients following acute myocardial infarction, ACE inhibitor therapy resulted in a significant reduction in risk of death (odds ratio: 0.83; 95% CI 0.71, 0.97), cardiovascular death (odds ratio: 0.82; 95% CI 0.69, 0.97), and SCD (odds ratio: 0.80; 95% CI 0.70, 0.92). The reduction in SCD risk seems therefore to be an important component of the survival benefit observed with ACE inhibitor therapy. A further systematic overview[36] of five long-term, randomized trials comparing ACE inhibitor treatment with placebo showed that ACE inhibitors lower rates of mortality, myocardial infarction, and hospital admission for heart failure in patients with LV dysfunction with or without a recent myocardial infarction, thus suggesting the use of ACE inhibitors in patients with LV dysfunction irrespective of the proximity to a myocardial infarction.

More recently, the HOPE trial[37,38] analyzed patients without LV dysfunction or heart failure who were at high risk of cardiovascular events: in this setting, administration of ramipril significantly affected the combined endpoint of death, myocardial infarction or stroke (serious arrhythmic events were also reduced). Finally, focusing on a low-risk population with stable coronary artery disease and no apparent heart failure, the EUROPA trial[39] showed that perindopril administration can reduce the risk of cardiovascular death, myocardial infarction or cardiac arrest.

**Table 5.3** Main prospective trials of angiotensin-converting enzyme inhibitors in prevention of mortality and SCD

| Acronym/title | No. patients | Follow-up | Endpoint | P | RRR (95% CI) |
|---|---|---|---|---|---|
| CONSENSUS/ Cooperative North Scandinavian Enalapril Survival Study (1987) | 253 | 188 days | Overall mortality | 0.003 | 27% (5% to 50%) |
| | | | SCD | >0.25 | 1% (–69% to 71%) |
| SOLVD/Effect of Enalapril on Survival in Patients with reduced LV ejection fractions and CHF (1991) | 2569 | 41.4 months | Cardiovascular mortality | <0.002 | 13% (3% to 24%) |
| | | | Overall mortality | <0.003 | 11% (2% to 21%) |
| | | | Death from arrhythmia without worsening CHF | N.S. | 7% (–18% to 31%) |
| SOLVD/Effect of Enalapril on Survival in Asymptomatic Patients with reduced LV ejection fractions (1992) | 4228 | 37.4 months | Overall mortality | 0.30 | 6% (–7% to 20%) |
| | | | Death from CHD | 0.12 | 11% (–4% to 25%) |
| | | | Death from arrhythmia without worsening CHF | N.S. | 8% (–18% to 34%) |
| V-HeFT II/Veterans Administration Cooperative Vasodilator-Heart Failure Trial (1991) | 804 | 42 months | Death from CHD | 0.016 | 19% (0 to 37%) |
| | | | SCD | 0.015 | 35% (6% to 65%) |
| | | | Overall mortality | 0.08 | 14% (–3% to 32%) |
| SAVE/Survival and Ventricular Enlargement Trial (1992) | 2231 | 42 months | Death from CHD | 0.014 | 20% (4% to 35%) |
| | | | SCD | N.S. | 16% (–13 to 46%) |
| | | | Overall mortality | 0.019 | 17% (3% to 31%) |
| AIRE/Acute Infarction Ramipril Efficacy Study (1993) | 2006 | 15 months | Overall mortality | 0.002 | 25% (10% to 41%) |
| GISSI-3/Gruppo Italiano per lo Studio della Sopravvivenza nell'Infarto Miocardico (1994) | 19 394 | 6 weeks | Combined endpoint (mortality and severe ventricular dysfunction) | 2P=0.009 | 8% (2% to 14%) |
| | | | Overall mortality | 2P=0.03 | 11% (1% to 21%) |
| SMILE/Survival of Myocardial Infarction Long-Term Evaluation (1995) | 1556 | 6 weeks | Combined endpoint (death or severe CHF) | 0.018 | 33% (6% to 60%) |
| | | | SCD | N.S. | 64% (–4% to 100%) |
| | | | Overall mortality | 0.17 | 22% (–10% to 53%) |
| TRACE/Trandolapril Cardiac Evaluation Study (1995) | 6676 | 24 to 50 months | Death from CHD | 0.001 | 22% (9% to 35%) |
| | | | SCD | 0.03 | 21% (0 to 42%) |
| | | | Overall mortality | 0.001 | 18% (7% to 29%) |

**Table 5.3** (Continued)

| Acronym/title | No. patients | Follow-up | Endpoint | *P* | RRR (95% CI) |
|---|---|---|---|---|---|
| ISIS-4/Fourth International Study of Infarct Survival (1995) | 58 050 | 5 weeks | Overall mortality | 2P=0.02 | 6% (1% to 12%) |
| CONSENSUS/Cooperative North Scandinavian Enalapril Survival Study (1987) | 253 | 188 days | Overall mortality | 0.003 | 27% (5% to 50%) |
| | | | SCD | >0.25 | 1% (−69% to 71%) |
| SOLVD/Effect of Enalapril on Survival in Patients with reduced left ventricular ejection fractions and congestive heart failure (1991) | 2569 | 41.4 months | Cardiovascular mortality | <0.002 | 13% (3% to 24%) |
| | | | Overall mortality | <0.003 | 11% (2% to 21%) |
| | | | Death from arrhythmia without worsening CHF | N.S. | 7% (−18% to 31%) |

CI=confidence interval; N.S.=not significant; RRR=relative risk reduction; SCD=sudden cardiac death; CHD=coronary heart disease; CHF=congestive heart failure

Based on this broad set of trials, at the present time, the ESC guidelines[19] recommend ACE inhibitors (class I) for primary prevention of SCD in patients with previous myocardial infarction, with or without LV dysfunction.

## ANGIOTENSIN RECEPTOR BLOCKER AGENTS

The potential antiarrhythmic effect of angiotensin receptor blocker agents (ARBs) has been explained in terms of AT1 receptor blockade leading to inhibition of the proarrhythmic effects of angiotensin II (decrease in intracellular resistance, increase in conduction velocity, and shortening of the refractory period of cardiac myocytes).[20] Selective blockade of AT1 receptors leaves stimulation of AT2 receptors unopposed. The effects of AT2 receptors are still unclear, but seem to be antiproliferative and opposed to those of AT1 receptors. ARBs also exert beneficial cardiovascular effects through neurohormonal and hemodynamic mechanisms.

The ELITE trial[40] compared losartan with captopril in elderly heart-failure patients: treatment with losartan was associated with a significant decrease in all-cause mortality (Table 5.4). The ELITE II study[41] enrolled a larger number of heart-failure patients but was unable to find any significant difference between losartan and captopril in terms of all-cause mortality or SCD. Similar results were obtained in the OPTIMAAL trial,[42] which included patients with acute myocardial infarction and heart failure, randomly assigned to losartan or captopril. The effects of adding an ARB to the standard therapy for heart failure were analyzed in the Val–HeFT trial.[43] Overall mortality was similar in the intervention and the placebo-controlled arms. Subgroup analysis suggested significant survival benefits from valsartan in patients not taking an ACE inhibitor. The LIFE study[44] compared losartan with atenolol

**Table 5.4** Main prospective trials of angiotensin II antagonists in prevention of mortality and SCD

| Acronym/title | No. patients | Follow-up | Endpoint | *P* | RRR (95% CI) |
|---|---|---|---|---|---|
| ELITE/Evaluation of Losartan in the Elderly Study (1997) | 722 | 48 weeks | Overall mortality | 0.035 | 44% (2% to 86%) |
| | | | SCD | <0.05 | 63% (3% to 100%) |
| ELITE II/Losartan Heart Failure Survival Study (2000) | 3152 | 555 days | Overall mortality | 0.16 | –11% (–28% to 5%) |
| | | | SCD or resuscitated cardiac arrest | 0.08 | –23% (–49% to 3%) |
| Val-HeFT/Valsartan Heart Failure Trial (2001) | 5010 | 23 months | Overall mortality | 0.80 | –2% (–13% to 10%) |
| OPTIMAAL/Optimal Trial in Myocardial Infarction with the Angiotensin II Antagonist Losartan (2002) | 5477 | 2.7 years | Overall mortality | 0.069 | –11% (–23% to 1%) |
| | | | SCD or resuscitated cardiac arrest | 0.072 | –18% (–37% to 2%) |
| LIFE/Losartan Intervention for Endpoint Reduction (2002) | 9193 | 4.8 years | Cardiovascular morbidity and mortality | 0.009 | 14% (4% to 24%) |
| CHARM/Candesartan in Heart Failure Assessment of Reduction in Mortality and Morbididy (2004) | 4576 | 40 months | Cardiovascular mortality | 0.005 | 13% (3% to 22%) |
| | | | Overall mortality | 0.018 | 10% (1% to 18%) |

CI = confidence interval; SCD = sudden cardiac death; RRR = relative risk reduction

as antihypertensive treatments: a significant reduction in the primary composite endpoint of cardiovascular morbidity and mortality was seen in the losartan arm.

In a meta-analysis[45] of 17 randomized, controlled trials comparing ARBs with either placebo or ACE inhibitors in patients with symptomatic heart failure, ARBs were not superior to controls in reducing all-cause mortality (odds ratio: 0.96; 95% CI 0.75, 1.23). Stratified analysis, however, showed a nonsignificant trend in benefit of ARBs over placebo in reducing mortality when an ARB was given in the absence of ACE inhibitor therapy. The combination therapy of ARBs and ACE inhibitors was superior to ACE inhibitors alone in reducing hospitalization, but not mortality.

By contrast, in the CHARM trial[46] candesartan appeared to reduce significantly all-cause mortality, cardiovascular death and heart-failure hospitalization in patients with chronic heart failure and LVEF of ≤40% when added to standard therapies including ACE inhibitors, beta-blockers and aldosterone antagonists. In a recent meta-analysis[47] of 24 trials, including the CHARM study, use of ARBs in patients with chronic heart failure was associated with reduced all-cause mortality (odds ratio 0.83; 95% CI 0.69, 1.00) as compared with placebo, but no difference was seen between ARBs and ACE inhibitors in terms of reduction in all-cause mortality and heart failure hospitalization. The combination therapy of ARBs and ACE inhibitors did not provide a significant reduction in all-cause mortality as compared with ACE inhibitors alone.

Taken together, the results of this series of randomized, multicenter trials do not seem to provide evidence that ARBs are superior to ACE inhibitors. However, use of ARBs may be suggested in patients who are intolerant of ACE inhibitors.

## STATINS

The influence of statins on clinical events is related to their pleiotropic effects. Their cholesterol-lowering and antioxidant properties help attenuate endothelial dysfunction, prevent plaque rupture in vascular walls, and inhibit platelet aggregation and thrombus formation. Statins also reduce the levels of C-reactive protein, and their anti-inflammatory properties could contribute to their plaque-stabilization effects. The antiarrhythmic effect of statin therapy can probably be attributed to a combination of these mechanisms.[20]

Many trials have shown significant reductions in all-cause mortality after statin therapy (Table 5.5). These benefits were mostly paralleled by reduced SCD, although few specific data on this endpoint were separately reported.

In the 4S study,[48] long-term treatment with simvastatin significantly reduced all-cause mortality in patients with coronary heart disease and hypercholesterolemia. In the LIPID trial,[49] pravastatin significantly reduced overall mortality and deaths from coronary heart disease in patients with a history of myocardial infarction or unstable angina showing a broad range of cholesterol levels. Similar benefits were found in the CARE trial[50] in patients with previous myocardial infarction and average low-density lipoprotein (LDL) levels.

The effects of statins in primary prevention of cardiovascular events have been analyzed in two randomized, placebo-controlled trials. The WOSCOPS trial evaluated the effects of pravastatin in patients with hypercholesterolemia and no history of coronary artery disease,[51] while AFCAPS/TexCAPS[52] focused on the use of lovastatin in a similar population without clinically evident cardiovascular disease, characterized by average total cholesterol and LDL levels accompanied by below-average high-density lipoprotein (HDL) levels. Both interventions led to significant reductions in the incidence of major cardiovascular events.

A meta-analysis of these first five trials[53] showed significant risk reduction benefits (with odds ratios of 0.68 for cardiovascular mortality and 0.87 for all-cause mortality in the two primary prevention trials, and 0.73 and 0.77, respectively, in the three secondary prevention trials).

Recently, the results of PROSPER[54] indicated that pravastatin can reduce mortality in elderly subjects at high risk of developing cardiovascular disease and stroke, suggesting that the benefits of statins extend into old age. The lipid-lowering component of ALLHAT (involving a subset of patients enrolled in this trial) was designed to assess whether pravastatin therapy can reduce all-cause mortality with respect to usual care in elderly, moderately hypercholesterolemic, hypertensive patients with at least one additional cardiovascular risk factor.[55] This substudy did not reveal any significant difference in all-cause mortality, although this negative result may be related to the unblinded nature of the study, the absence of a placebo arm, and the large cross-over of higher-risk patients from usual care to the statin arm.[56] In ASCOT-LLA,[57] atorvastatin therapy showed potential for primary prevention of cardiovascular events in patients with multiple cardiovascular risk factors; there was also a nonsignificant trend toward reduced all-cause mortality.

For patients with acute coronary syndrome, the MIRACL study[58] showed that when lipid-lowering therapy with atorvastatin (80 mg daily) is initiated 24–96 h after

**Table 5.5** Main prospective trials of statins in prevention of mortality and SCD

| Acronym/title | No. patients | Follow-up | Endpoint | *P* | RRR (95% CI) |
|---|---|---|---|---|---|
| 4S/Scandinavian Simvastatin Survival Study (1994) | 4444 | 5.4 years | Death from CHD | <0.001 | 38% (19% to 56%) |
| | | | All-cause deaths | 0.0003 | 27% (12% to 43%) |
| WOSCOPS/West of Scotland Coronary Prevention Study Group (1995) | 6595 | 4.9 years | Death from CHD or nonfatal MI | <0.001 | 31% (16% to 46%) |
| | | | All-cause deaths | 0.051 | 25% (3% to 47%) |
| CARE/Cholesterol and Recurrent Events trial (1996) | 4159 | 5 years | Death from CHD or nonfatal MI | 0.003 | 23% (8% to 38%) |
| | | | All-cause deaths | 0.37 | 9% (−10% to 27%) |
| LIPID/Long-Term Intervention with Pravastatin in Ischaemic Disease (1998) | 9014 | 6.1 years | Death from CHD | <0.001 | 25% (12% to 38%) |
| | | | All-cause deaths | <0.001 | 21% (12% to 31%) |
| AFCAPS TexCAPS/ Air Force/Texas Coronary Atherosclerosis Prevention Study (1998) | 6605 | 5.2 years | Acute major coronary event (MI, unstable angina or SCD) | <0.001 | 36% (24% to 49%) |
| MIRACL/Myocardial Ischemia Reduction with Aggressive Cholesterol Lowering study (2001) | 3086 | 16 weeks | Composite of death, nonfatal MI, cardiac arrest, symptomatic myocardial ischemia | 0.48 | 12% (−3% to 37%) |
| HPS/Heart Protection Study (2002) | 20 536 | 5 years | Death from CHD | 0.0005 | 14% (5% to 24%) |
| | | | All-cause deaths | 0.0003 | 13% (7% to 20%) |
| PROSPER/Pravastatin in Elderly Individuals at Risk of Vascular Disease (2002) | 5804 | 3.2 years | Composite of death from CHD, nonfatal MI, stroke | 0.014 | 13% (2% to 24%) |
| ALLHAT-LLT/ Antihypertensive and Lipid-Lowering Treatment to Prevent Heart Attack Trial (2002) | 10 355 | 4.8 years | Death from CHD | 0.16 | 0% (−22% to 22%) |
| | | | All-cause deaths | 0.88 | 2% (−9% to 12%) |
| ASCOT/Anglo-Scandinavian Cardiac Outcomes Trial–Lipid Lowering Arm (2003) | 10 305 | 3.3 years | Death from CHD or nonfatal MI | 0.0005 | 37% (17% to 57%) |
| | | | All-cause deaths | 0.1649 | 12% (−6% to 30%) |
| PACT/Pravastatin in Acute Coronary Treatment (2004) | 3408 | 4 weeks | Composite of death, recurrence of MI or unstable angina | N.S. | 6% (−11% to 24%) |
| | | | SCD | N.S. | 20% (−70% to 100%) |

**Table 5.5** (Continued)

| Acronym/title | No. patients | Follow-up | Endpoint | *P* | RRR (95% CI) |
|---|---|---|---|---|---|
| PROVE IT-TIMI 22/ Pravastatin or Atorvastatin Evaluation and Infection Therapy–Thrombolysis in Myocardial Infarction 22 (2004) | 4162 | 24 months | Composite of all-cause death, MI, unstable angina, revascularization, stroke | 0.005 | 15% (5% to 25%) |
| TNT/Treating New Targets Trial (2005) | 10001 | 4.9 years | Acute major coronary event (death from CHD, nonfatal MI, cardiac arrest, stroke) | <0.001 | 18% (7% to 29%) |
| | | | All-cause deaths | 0.92 | 0 (–16% to 16%) |

CHD = coronary heart disease; MI = myocardial infarction; CI = confidence interval; SCD = sudden cardiac death; RRR = relative risk reduction

an acute coronary event, it can reduce ischemic recurrences in the first 16 weeks. In the PACT trial, initiation of pravastatin within 24 h of an acute coronary event was found to be safe, with a favorable, albeit nonsignificant, trend toward a reduction in the primary composite endpoint of death, recurrence of myocardial infarction or readmission to hospital for unstable angina within 30 days of the acute coronary event.[59]

In a meta-analysis of 15 lipid trials,[60] statin therapy significantly reduced relative risk (RR) of coronary events by 27% (95% CI 23, 32%), cardiovascular disease mortality by 22% (95% CI 16, 27%) and all-cause death by 15% (95% CI 11, 19%). Recently, a further meta-analysis of 10 outcome trials of statins[61] showed that statin therapy reduces major coronary events by 27% (95% CI 23, 30%), stroke by 18% (95% CI 10, 25%), and all-cause mortality by 15% (95% CI 8, 21%). Coronary events were reduced by 23% (95% CI 18, 29%) in pravastatin trials and 29% (95% CI 25, 33%) in five trials with other statins.

The Heart Protection Study[62] and PROVE IT-TIMI 22 (Pravastatin or Atorvastatin Evaluation and Infection Therapy – Thrombolysis in Myocardial Infarction)[63] showed not only that patients with cardiovascular disease and very high risk of coronary heart disease had substantial reductions in all-cause and cardiovascular mortality with statin therapy, but also that these survival benefits were accompanied by reductions in LDL values to well below 100 mg/dl, suggesting that this level does not constitute a threshold below which no further benefit from statins can be achieved.

Based on the findings of HPS and PROVE IT, in 2004 the National Cholesterol Education Program Adult Treatment Panel III guidelines[56] suggested a LDL goal of <70 mg/dl for high-risk patients, and strongly recommended the same target for very-high-risk patients, defined as patients with established cardiovascular disease plus either 1) multiple major risk factors (especially diabetes); or 2) severe and poorly controlled risk factors; or 3) multiple risk factors of the metabolic syndrome; or 4) acute coronary syndromes. Recently, the TNT study[64] evaluated the safety and efficacy of lowering LDL values to <100 mg/dl in patients with stable coronary artery disease treated with atorvastatin. Patients were randomly assigned to double-blind therapy and received either 10 or 80 mg atorvastatin per day. The intensive lipid-lowering therapy with 80 mg atorvastatin per day significantly reduced the occurrence of a first major cardiovascular event, defined as death from coronary heart disease, nonfatal myocardial infarction, resuscitation after cardiac arrest, or stroke. There was no difference between the two treatment groups in all-cause mortality. However, the cardiovascular benefits of this aggressive lipid-lowering therapy were associated with a greater incidence of elevated aminotransferase levels. Anyway, these data confirm and extend the evidence that lowering LDL cholesterol to levels below those currently recommended can bring additional cardiovascular benefits.

## OMEGA-3 FATTY ACIDS

Omega-3 fatty acids may provide cardiovascular health benefits due to several effects. These include decrease in very-low-density lipoprotein (VLDL) and thereby in plasma triglyceride levels, improvement in endothelial function, cell membrane stabilization, platelet aggregation inhibition, suppression of smooth muscle cell proliferation and prevention of calcium overload.[20]

As can be seen from Table 5.6, several clinical trials support the concept that omega-3 fatty acids can reduce the risk of overall and cardiovascular mortality in patients with coronary heart disease.[65–71] In the GISSI-Prevention study,[68] the use of omega-3 fatty acids significantly reduced the primary combined endpoint of death, nonfatal myocardial infarction and nonfatal stroke, with a benefit attributable to a decrease in the risk of overall and cardiovascular death. In a meta-analysis of 11 trials,[72] comparing dietary or nondietary intake of n-3 fatty acids with placebo or control diet in patients with coronary heart disease, the estimated risk ratio was 0.7 for fatal myocardial infarction and 0.8 for overall mortality; in five of these trials, SCD was associated with a risk ratio of 0.7. A further meta-analysis[73] suggests that the supplementation with n-3 fatty acids in patients with coronary heart disease significantly reduces the incidence of death from all causes by 16% (relative risk 0.8) and the incidence of death due to fatal myocardial infarction by 24% (relative risk 0.7).

Recently, a systematic review[74] of randomized, controlled trials comparing any lipid-lowering intervention with placebo or usual diet underlined significant risk-reduction benefit from statins and n-3 fatty acids (with risk ratios of 0.78 for cardiovascular mortality and 0.87 for all-cause mortality for statins, and 0.68 and 0.77, respectively, for n-3 fatty acids).

Based on results of clinical trials, the ESC guidelines suggest intake of omega-3 fatty acids (class IIa recommendation) for primary prevention of SCD in patients with previous myocardial infarction.[19]

## MAGNESIUM

Magnesium can suppress enhanced automaticity and triggered activity, thus preventing torsade de pointes, regardless of serum magnesium concentration. Hypomagnesemia is a potent trigger of ventricular arrhythmia, and appropriate substitution of this electrolyte can prevent arrhythmia.

**Table 5.6** Main prospective trials of omega-3 fatty acids in prevention of mortality and SCD

| Acronym/title | No. patients | Follow-up | Endpoint | *P* | RRR (95% CI) |
|---|---|---|---|---|---|
| DART/Diet and Reinfarction Trial (1989) | 2033 | 2 years | Nonfatal MI | N.S. | –50% (–103% to 3%) |
| | | | Cardiovascular mortality | <0.01 | 32% (10% to 55%) |
| | | | Overall mortality | <0.05 | 27% (6% to 49%) |
| Indian/Indian Experiment of Infarct Survival (1997) | 404 | 1 year | Nonfatal MI | <0.01 | 48% (10% to 87%) |
| | | | Fatal MI | <0.05 | 36% (–19% to 91%) |
| | | | SCD | N.S. | 76% (2% to 100%) |
| | | | Overall mortality | <0.05 | 48% (5% to 90%) |
| Lyon/Lyon Diet Heart Study (1999) | 605 | 46 months | Nonfatal MI | 0.01 | 70% (28% to 100%) |
| | | | Fatal MI | 0.01 | 71% (22% to 100%) |
| | | | Overall mortality | 0.03 | 46% (–1% to 92%) |
| GISSI/Prevenzione/ Gruppo Italiano per lo Studio della Sopravvivenza nell'infarto (1999) | 11 324 | 3.5 years | Fatal MI | <0.05 | 19% (3% to 35%) |
| | | | SCD | 0.010 | 24% (4% to 44%) |
| | | | Overall mortality | <0.05 | 14% (3% to 24%) |

CI=confidence interval; SCD=sudden cardiac death; RRR=relative risk reduction; MI=myocardial infarction

Although the electrophysiologic properties of magnesium can explain its antiarrhythmic effect, data from trials (Table 5.7) on magnesium infusion yielded contradictory results in patients without hypomagnesemia.[33,75,76] In the MAGIC trial,[76] early administration of magnesium in high-risk patients with acute myocardial infarction had no effect on 30-day mortality. Therefore, the role of magnesium in prevention of SCD is still unclear.

## CONCLUSIONS

SCD may occur in many different types of heart diseases, and even in apparently healthy subjects, as a result of the complex interaction of many factors, which may be variously related (in terms of proximity and causation) to the electrical event (i.e., ventricular fibrillation). Therefore, it is not surprising that some pharmacologic interactions, initially thought to be devoid of what is usually considered as a true 'antiarrhythmic' effect, may indeed reduce SCD. These agents have usually, in variable degrees, effects on factors involved in the processes that lead to ischemia and infarction, effects on autonomic nervous system modulation and sympathetic activation, and direct or indirect effects on cardiac membrane electrical properties. The evidence that some agents have favorable effects on sudden death is of great value for improving our attempts to reduce the overall burden of sudden death, especially when dealing with populations at relatively low risk of sudden death. Moreover, in patients at higher risk of SCD, these agents may be associated with other interventions (i.e., revascularization procedures, implantable devices) in an attempt to obtain

**Table 5.7** Main prospective trials of magnesium in prevention of mortality and SCD

| Acronym/title | No. patients | Follow-up | Endpoint | *P* | RRR (95% CI) |
|---|---|---|---|---|---|
| LIMIT-2/Leicester Intravenous Magnesium Intervention Trial (1992) | 2316 | 28 days | All-cause death | 0.03 | 24% (2% to 47%) |
| ISIS-4/Fourth International Study of Infarct Survival (1995) | 58 050 | 5 weeks | All-cause death | 2P=0.07 | −6% (−11% to 0) |
| MAGIC/Magnesium in Coronaries Trial (2002) | 6213 | 30 days | All-cause death | 0.96 | −1% (−12% to 11%) |

CI=confidence interval; RRR=relative risk reduction

an additive or, even, a synergetic effect. The effects of a pharmacologic agent on SCD are usually evaluated in parallel with the effects on overall mortality, which continues to be an undisputed, although crude, endpoint. However evaluation of the specific effect of an agent on SCD continues to be of both clinical and speculative interest, since new approaches to improve patient outcome might be identified by such analysis and be considered for further investigation.

## REFERENCES

1. Myerburg RJ, Interian AJ, Mitrani RM et al. Frequency of sudden cardiac death and profiles of risk. Am J Cardiol 1997; 80: 10F–19F.
2. Josephson M, Wellens HJJ. Implantable defibrillators and sudden cardiac death. Circulation 2004; 109: 2685–91.
3. Zheng ZJ, Croft JB, Giles WH et al. Sudden cardiac death in the United States, 1989 to 1998. Circulation 2001; 104: 2158–63.
4. Bardy GH, Lee KL, Mark DB et al for the Sudden Cardiac Death in Heart Failure Trial (SCD-HeFT) Investigators. Amiodarone or an implantable cardioverter-defibrillator for congestive heart failure. N Engl J Med 2005; 352: 225–37.
5. Lopez-Sendon J, Swedberg K, McMurray J et al. Expert consensus document on beta-adrenergic receptor blockers. Eur Heart J 2004; 25: 1341–62.
6. CIBIS Investigators and Committees. A randomized trial of β-blockade in heart failure. The cardiac insufficiency bisoprolol study (CIBIS). Circulation 1994; 90: 1765–73.
7. CIBIS II Investigators and Committees. The cardiac insufficiency bisoprolol study II (CIBIS II): a randomised trial. Lancet 1999; 353: 9–13.
8. MERIT-HF Study Group. Effect of metoprolol CR/XL in chronic heart failure: metoprolol CR/XL randomised intervention trial in congestive heart failure (MERIT HF). Lancet 1999; 353: 2001–7.
9. Packer M, Coats AJS, Fowler MB et al. Effect of carvedilol on survival in severe chronic heart failure. N Engl J Med 2001; 344: 1651–8.
10. The Beta-Blocker Evaluation of Survival Trial Investigators. A trial of the beta-blocker bucindolol in patients with advanced chronic heart failure. N Engl J Med 2001; 344: 1659–67.

11. The CAPRICORN Investigators. Effect of carvedilol on outcome after myocardial infarction in patients with left-ventricular dysfunction: the CAPRICORN randomized trial. Lancet 2001; 357: 1385–90.
12. Poole-Wilson PA, Swedberg K, Cleland JGF et al. Comparison of carvedilol and metoprolol on clinical outcomes in patients with chronic heart failure in the Carvedilol or Metoprolol European Trial (COMET): randomized controlled trial. Lancet 2003; 362: 7–13.
13. Lechat P, Packer M, Chalon S et al. Clinical effects of β-adrenergic blockade in chronic heart failure. A meta-analysis of double-blind, placebo-controlled, randomized trials. Circulation 1998; 98: 1184–91.
14. Brophy JM, Joseph L, Rouleau JL. β-Blockers in congestive heart failure. Ann Intern Med 2001; 134: 550–60.
15. Lee S, Spencer A. Beta-blockers to reduce mortality in patients with systolic dysfunction: a meta-analysis. J Fam Pract 2001; 50: 499–504.
16. Cleophas TJ, Zwinderman AH. Beta-blockers and heart failure: meta-analysis of mortality trials. Int J Clin Pharmacol Ther 2001; 39: 383–8.
17. Freemantle N, Cleland JG, Young P et al. Beta-blocked after myocardial infarction: systematic review and meta regression analysis. BMJ 2001; 318: 1730–7.
18. Dulin BR, Haas SJ, Abraham WT et al. Do elderly systolic heart failure patients benefit from beta blockers to the same extent as the non-elderly? Meta-analysis of >12 000 patients in large-scale clinical trials. Am J Cardiol 2005; 95: 896–98.
19. Priori SG, Aliot E, Blomstrom-Lundqvist C et al. Task Force on Sudden Cardiac Death of the European Society of Cardiology. Europace 2002; 4: 3–18.
20. Alberte C, Zipes DP. Use of non-antiarrhythmic drugs for prevention of sudden cardiac death. J Cardiovasc Electrophysiol 2003; 14: S87–S95.
21. MacFayden RJ, Barr CS, Struthers AD. Aldosterone blockade reduces vascular collagen turnover, improves heart rate variability and reduces early morning rise in heart rate in heart failure patients. Cardiovasc Res 1997; 35: 30–34.
22. Farquharson CA, Struthers AD. Aldosterone induces acute endothelial dysfunction in vivo in humans: evidence for an aldosterone-induced vasculopathy. Clin Sci (Lond) 2002; 103: 425–31.
23. Pitt B, Zannad F, Remme WJ et al. The effect of spironolactone on morbidity and mortality in patients with severe heart failure. N Engl J Med 1999; 341: 709–17.
24. Pitt B, Remme W, Zannad F et al. Eplerenone, a selective aldosterone blocker, in patients with left ventricular dysfunction after myocardial infarction. N Engl J Med 2003; 348: 1309–21.
25. The CONSENSUS Trial Study Group. Effects of enalapril on mortality in severe congestive heart failure. N Engl J Med 1987; 316: 1429–35.
26. The SOLVD Investigators. Effect of enalapril on survival in patients with reduced left ventricular ejection fractions and congestive heart failure. N Engl J Med 1991; 325: 293–302.
27. The SOLVD Investigators. Effect of enalapril on mortality and the development of heart failure in asymptomatic patients with reduced left ventricular ejection fractions. N Engl J Med 1992; 327: 685–91.
28. Cohn JN, Johnson G, Ziesche S et al. A comparison of enalapril with hydralazine-isosorbide dinitrate in the treatment of chronic congestive heart failure. N Engl J Med 1991; 325: 303–10.
29. Pfeffer MA, Braunwald E, Moyè LA et al. Effect of captopril on mortality and morbidity in patients with left ventricular dysfunction after myocardial infarction. N Engl J Med 1992; 327: 669–77.
30. The AIRE Investigators. Effect of ramipril on mortality and morbidity of survivors of acute myocardial infarction with clinical evidence of heart failure. Lancet 1993; 342: 821–28.
31. Kober L, Torp-Pedersen C, Carlsen JE et al. A clinical trial of the angiotensin converting enzyme inhibitor trandolapril in patients with left ventricular dysfunction after myocardial infarction. N Engl J Med 1995; 333: 1670–6.

32. The GISSI-3 Investigators. GISSI-3: effects of lisinopril and transdermal glyceryl trinitrate singly and together on 6-week mortality and ventricular function after acute myocardial infarction. Lancet 1994; 343: 1115–22.
33. The ISIS-4 Investigators. ISIS-4: a randomized factorial trial assessing early oral captopril, oral mononitrate, and intravenous magnesium sulphate in 58 050 patients with suspected acute myocardial infarction. Lancet 1995; 345: 669–85.
34. Ambrosioni E, Borghi C, Magnani B et al. The effect of angiotensin converting enzyme inhibitor zofenopril on mortality and morbidity after anterior myocardial infarction. N Engl J Med 1995; 332: 80–5.
35. Domanski MJ, Exner DV, Borkowf CB et al. Effect of angiotensin converting enzyme inhibition on sudden cardiac death in patients following acute myocardial infarction. A meta-analysis of randomized clinical trials. J Am Coll Cardiol 1999; 33: 598–604.
36. Flather MD, Yusuf S, Kober L et al. Long-term ACE-inhibitor therapy in patients with heart failure or left-ventricular dysfunction: a systematic overview of data from individual patients. Lancet 2000; 355: 1575–81.
37. The HOPE Investigators. Effects of an angiotensin converting enzyme inhibitor, ramipril, on cardiovascular events in high-risk patients. N Engl J Med 2000; 342: 145–53.
38. Teo KK, Mitchell LB, Pogue J et al. Effect of ramipril in reducing sudden deaths and nonfatal cardiac arrests in high risk individuals without heart failure or left ventricular dysfunction. Circulation 2004; 110: 1413–17.
39. The EUROPA Investigators. Efficacy of perindopril in reduction of cardiovascular events among patients with stable coronary artery disease: randomised, double-blind, placebo-controlled, multicentre trial (the EUROPA study). Lancet 2003; 362: 782–88.
40. Pitt B, Segal R, Martinez FA et al. Randomised trial of losartan versus captopril in patients over 65 with heart failure (Evaluation of Losartan in the Elderly study, ELITE). Lancet 1997; 349: 747–52.
41. Pitt B, Poole-Wilson PA, Segal R et al. Effect of losartan compared with captopril on mortality in patients with symptomatic heart failure: randomised trial – the Losartan Heart Failure Survival Study ELITE II. Lancet 2000; 355: 1582–87.
42. Dickstein K, Kjekshus J, and the OPTIMAAL study group. Effects of losartan and captopril on mortality and morbidity in high-risk patients after acute myocardial infarction: the OPTIMAAL randomised trial. Lancet 2002; 360: 752–60.
43. Cohn JN, Tognoni G, for the Valsartan Heart Failure Trial Investigators. A randomized trial of the angiotensin receptor blocker valsartan in chronic heart failure. N Engl J Med 2001; 345: 1667–75.
44. Dahlof B, Devereux RB, Kjeldsen SE et al. Cardiovascular morbidity and mortality in the Losartan Intervention for Endpoint reduction in hypertension study (LIFE): a randomised trial against atenolol. Lancet 2002; 359: 995–1003.
45. Jong P, Demers C, McKelvie RS et al. Angiotensin receptor blockers in heart failure: meta-analysis of randomized controlled trials. J Am Coll Cardiol 2002; 39: 463–70.
46. Young JB, Dunlap ME, Pfeffer MA et al. Mortality and morbidity reduction with candesartan in patients with chronic heart failure and left ventricular systolic dysfunction: results of the CHARM low-left ventricular ejection fraction trials. Circulation 2004; 110: 2618–26.
47. Lee VC, Rhew DC, Dylan M et al. Meta-analysis: angiotensin-receptor blockers in chronic heart failure and high-risk acute myocardial infarction. Ann Intern Med 2004; 141: 693–704.
48. Scandinavian Simvastatin Survival Study Group. Randomised trial of cholesterol lowering in 4444 patients with coronary heart disease: the Scandinavian Simvastatin Survival Study (4S). Lancet 1994; 344: 1383–89.
49. The LIPID study group. Prevention of cardiovascular events and death with pravastatin in patients with coronary heart disease and a broad range of initial cholesterol levels. N Engl J Med 1998; 339: 1349–57.
50. Sacks FM, Pfeffer MA, Lemuel AM et al. The effect of pravastatin on coronary events after myocardial infarction in patients with average cholesterol levels. N Engl J Med 1996; 335: 1001–9.

51. Shepherd J, Cobbe S, Ford I et al. Prevention of coronary heart disease with pravastatin in men with hypercholesterolemia. N Engl J Med 1995; 333: 1301–7.
52. Downs JR, Clearfield M, Weis S et al. Primary prevention of acute coronary events with lovastatin in men and women with average cholesterol levels: results of AFCAPS/TexCAPS. Air Force/Texas Coronary Atherosclerosis Prevention Study. JAMA 1998; 279: 1615–22.
53. LaRosa JC, He J, Vupputuri S. Effects of statins on risk of coronary disease: a meta-analysis of randomized controlled trials. JAMA 1999; 282: 2340–6.
54. Shepherd J, Blauw GJ, Murphy MB et al, PROSPER study group. Pravastatin in elderly individuals at risk of vascular disease (PROSPER): a randomized controlled trial. PROspective Study of Pravastatin in the Elderly at Risk. Lancet 2002; 360: 1623–30.
55. ALLHAT Collaborative Research Group. The Antihypertensive and Lipid-Lowering Treatment to Prevent Heart Attack Trial. Major outcomes in moderately hypercholesterolemic, hypertensive patients randomized to pravastatin vs usual care: the Antihypertensive and Lipid-Lowering Treatment to Prevent Heart Attack Trial. JAMA 2002; 288: 2998–3007.
56. Grundy SM, Cleeman JI, Merz CNB et al. Implications of recent clinical trials for the National Cholesterol Education Program Adult Treatment Panel III guidelines. J Am Coll Cardiol 2004; 44: 720–32.
57. Sever PS, Dahlof B, Poulter NR et al. ASCOT investigators. Prevention of coronary and stroke events with atorvastatin in hypertensive patients who have average or lower-than-average cholesterol concentrations, in the Anglo-Scandinavian Cardiac Outcomes Trial-Lipid Lowering Arm (ASCOT-LLA): a multicentre randomised controlled trial. Lancet 2003; 361: 1149–58.
58. Schwartz GG, Olsson AG, Ezekowitz MD et al. Effects of atorvastatin on early recurrent ischemic events in acute coronary syndromes. JAMA 2001; 285: 1711–18.
59. Thompson PL, Meredith I, Amarena J et al. Effect of pravastatin compared with placebo initiated 24 hours of onset of acute myocardial infarction or unstable angina: the Pravastatin in Acute Coronary Treatment (PACT) trial. Am Heart J 2004; 148: E1–E8.
60. Vrecer M, Turk S, Drinovec J et al. Use of statins in primary and secondary prevention of coronary heart disease and ischemic stroke. Meta-analysis of randomized trials. Int J Clin Pharmacol Ther 2003; 41: 567–77.
61. Cheung BMY, Lauder IJ, Lau C et al. Meta-analysis of large randomized controlled trials to evaluate the impact of statins on cardiovascular outcomes. Br J Clin Pharmacol 2004; 57: 640–51.
62. Heart Protection Study Collaborative Group. MRC/BHF Heart Protection Study of cholesterol lowering with simvastatin in 20 536 high-risk individuals: a randomised placebo-controlled trial. Lancet 2002; 360: 7–22.
63. Cannon CP, Braunwald E, McCabe CH et al, for the Pravastatin or Atorvastatin Evaluation and Infection Therapy – Thrombolysis in Myocardial Infarction 22 Investigators. Comparison of intensive and moderate lipid lowering with statins after acute coronary syndromes. N Engl J Med 2004; 350: 1495–1504.
64. LaRosa JC, Grundy SM, Waters DD et al for the Treating to New Targets (TNT) Investigators. Intensive lipid lowering with atorvastatin in patients with stable coronary disease. N Engl J Med 2005; 352: 1425–35.
65. Albert CM, Hennekens CH, O'Donnell CJ et al. Fish consumption and risk of sudden cardiac death. JAMA 1998; 279: 23–8.
66. Siscovick DS, Raghunathan TE, King I et al. Dietary intake and cell membrane levels of long-chain n-3 polyunsaturated fatty acids and the risk of primary cardiac arrest. JAMA 1995; 274: 1363–7.
67. De Lorgeril M, Salen P, Martin J et al. Mediterranean diet, traditional risk factors and the rate of cardiovascular complications after myocardial infarction. Circulation 1999; 99: 779–85.
68. GISSI-Prevenzione Investigators. Dietary supplementation with n-3 polyunsaturated fatty acids and vitamin E after myocardial infarction: results of the GISSI-Prevenzione trial. Lancet 1999; 354: 447–55.

69. Burr ML, Fehily AM, Gilbert JF et al. Effects of changes in fat, fish and fibre intakes on death and myocardial reinfarction: diet and reinfarction trial (DART). Lancet 1989; 2: 757–61.
70. Singh RB, Niaz MA, Sharma JP et al. Randomized, double-blind, placebo-controlled trial of fish oil and mustard oil in patients with suspected acute myocardial infarction: the Indian experiment of infarct survival–4. Cardiovasc Drugs Ther 1997; 11: 485–91.
71. Johansen O, Brekke M, Seljeflot I et al. n-3 fatty acids do not prevent restenosis after coronary angioplasty: results from the CART study. J Am Coll Cardiol 1999; 33: 1619–26.
72. Bucher HC, Hengstler P, Schindler C et al. n-3 polyunsaturated fatty acids in coronary heart disease: a meta-analysis of randomized controlled trials. Am J Med 2002; 112: 298–304.
73. Yzebe D, Lievre M. Fish oils in the care of coronary heart disease patients: a meta-analysis of randomized controlled trials. Fundam Clin Pharmacol 2004; 18: 581–92.
74. Studer M, Briel M, Leimenstoll B et al. Effect of different antilipidemic agents and diets on mortality. Arch Intern Med 2005; 165: 725–30.
75. Woods KL, Fletcher S, Roffe C et al. Intravenous magnesium sulphate in suspected acute myocardial infarction: results of the second Leicester Intravenous Magnesium Intervention Trial (LIMIT 2). Lancet 1992; 339: 1553–8.
76. Magnesium in Coronaries (MAGIC) trial investigators. Early administration of intravenous magnesium to high-risk patients with acute myocardial infarction in the Magnesium in Coronaries (MAGIC) Trial: a randomised controlled trial. Lancet 2002; 360: 1189–96.

# 6

# Heart failure and sudden cardiac death: an unsolved problem

Benjamin J Rhee, Jeanne E Poole and Gust H Bardy

## INTRODUCTION

Sudden cardiac death (SCD) accounts for 50% of cases of cardiovascular mortality in the USA and other industrialized countries.[1] An estimated 335 000 Americans die of coronary artery disease (CAD) each year, chiefly because of cardiac arrest due to ventricular arrhythmia.[2] In Europe, 400 000 deaths annually are attributed to SCD.[3] Despite improvement in age-adjusted mortality, cardiovascular disease remains the main cause of death in the USA.[4] In many cases, SCD is the first manifestation of CAD. Approximately 85–90% of SCD are due to a first arrhythmic event. The remaining 10–15% are due to recurrent events.[5]

The risk of SCD for patients with heart failure (HF) is elevated 6-9-fold over the general US population, even when compared with survivors of myocardial infarction (MI).[2] In spite of efforts to raise the public in awareness of SCD and basic cardiopulmonary resuscitation (CPR), advances in emergency medical services, increased availability of automated external defibrillators, and novel treatment modalities such as induced hypothermia, survival rates remain dismally poor, with an estimated 1–5% expected to survive to hospital discharge.[6–8] Implantable cardioverter-defibrillators (ICDs) were first used clinically in the 1980s, and the devices matured rapidly during the early 1990s. Multiple trials have now been completed that have demonstrated their efficacy in both primary and secondary prevention of SCD in patients with HF.

## EPIDEMIOLOGY

There are an estimated 5 million patients living with HF in the USA currently, and this number is increasing annually. Each year, 550 000 new cases are diagnosed.[2] An estimated 260 000 Americans die as a result of HF annually.[2] The overall prevalence of HF varies considerably by age, increasing to 10% in those over 75 years of age.[2] Importantly, there may be several million people with asymptomatic left ventricular dysfunction who have yet to be identified.[9] Age-adjusted 5-year mortality rates in the Framingham cohort in men and women with HF are 59% and 45% respectively,[10] and individuals with advanced HF have higher mortality rates.[11] Put differently, review of the data revealed that the prognosis for newly diagnosed HF patients requiring hospitalization was that one-half would die within 2–3 years after the index admission.[10]

While HF is usually a chronic disease characterized by progressive loss of ventricular function and frequent decompensation, SCD is not necessarily an event characterized by progressive worsening of symptoms. Most HF victims of SCD do not have advanced NYHA class IV HF. Many are relatively young, with only mild to moderate (NYHA classes I–III) HF symptoms, even including survivors of MI.[12]

## PATHOPHYSIOLOGY

Most SCD in HF patients is due to ventricular tachycardia (VT) or ventricular fibrillation (VF).[13] In severe HF, bradyarrhythmia may also occur, and some sudden deaths in HF patients may also be due to acute MI, pulmonary embolism, or stroke. The pathophysiologic mechanism that lowers the threshold for ectopy and possible fatal arrhythmia is probably multifactorial.

A number of factors have been characterized as contributing to the development of arrhythmia. These include electrolyte abnormalities, such as hypokalemia, hypomagnesemia, and ischemia; hypoxia/acidosis; drug abnormalities, including cardiac toxins and drug interactions; and autonomic fluctuations. There are a number of clinical conditions that predispose the heart to SCD as well, including CAD, ventricular scar, left ventricular hypertrophy (LVH), inflammatory and infiltrative disorders, and congenital abnormalities, such as ion channel defects or accessory pathways.

The complex syndrome that comprises HF involves a number of maladaptive molecular and cellular responses to perceived cardiac injury. These responses ultimately result in compensatory anatomic remodeling of the heart as well as disturbances in the heart's electrical activity. It is estimated that as many as 15% of all HF patients, and over 30% with moderate-to-severe symptoms, have inter- and intraventricular conduction delays with QRS duration greater than 120 ms, a condition that may result in mechanical ventricular dyssynchrony.[14] Ventricular dyssynchrony contributes to mitral valve dysfunction and reduced pumping efficiency, which in turn promotes further progressive left ventricular dysfunction and worsened HF symptoms. Ventricular dyssynchrony has also been associated with an increased risk of SCD.[15]

Although any single mechanism may not trigger SCD, combinations of factors may push a patient over the threshold for VT/VF and cardiac arrest. Chronic infarct areas and acute lesions have been demonstrated to have a strong association with SCD. Patients with other causes of HF than ischemic heart disease may have nonspecific changes, such as diffuse interstitial fibrosis and hypertrophy, which may alter the electrophysiologic properties of the myocardium.

## PREVENTING SCD

Medical therapy to improve HF has dramatically improved over the past decades. As understanding of the mechanisms of pathophysiology evolved, effective medical therapies improved mortality and quality of life. Angiotensin-converting enzyme (ACE) inhibitors, beta-blockers, and diuretics have become the mainstays of pharmacologic therapy. As the conception of HF evolved from that of a hemodynamic process to a neurohormonal one as well, additional agents such as spironolactone and angiotensin receptor blockers (ARB) were added to the armamentarium, further improving quality of life in HF patients and decreasing overall mortality, including death due to cardiac arrhythmia.

Medical therapy for preventing SCD in heart failure patients has focused on beta-blockers and amiodarone. Beta-blockers have been extensively studied for prevention of SCD in HF patients. Generally, all-cause mortality has been used as the primary endpoint, and, in patients, there certainly has been debate over how best to classify deaths: arrhythmic, pump failure, or other. Additionally, it is clear that the severity of HF affects the relative contribution of each potential cause to overall mortality. Nonetheless, the mortality data are clear. Beta-blockers have been studied in multiple randomized, placebo-controlled studies and have consistently demonstrated significant reduction in all-cause mortality.[16–22] These trials evaluated various beta-blockers, including metoprolol succinate, bisoprolol, and carvedilol, all of which were shown to reduce all-cause mortality in patients with HF by about 32–35%. Further insight was gained from the MERIT-HF and CIBIS II trials, which showed a reduction in risk of SCD of 41% ($P$=0.0002) and 44% ($P$=0.0011), respectively.[23,24] These findings evaluated the mortality benefit seen in beta-blockers in addition to ACE inhibitors. In fact, the benefit of beta blockade in HF patients is so profound that both US and European guidelines now state that beta-blockers are mandatory for the treatment of all patients with stable, mild, moderate, or severe HF. In addition, emerging data suggest that beta-blockers should be considered as first-line therapy in HF patients, even prior to initiation of ACE inhibitors.[25,26]

Amiodarone has also been investigated as a potential treatment to reduce SCD in HF patients. Despite limited understanding of its pharmacology, it has become a widely used agent for management of both atrial fibrillation and VT. Two pivotal trials evaluating its use in HF patients showed conflicting survival results, but demonstrated intriguing, unexpected findings. The Grupo de Estudio de la Sobrevida la Insuffiencia Cardiaca en Argentina (GESICA) trial evaluated 516 patients with ejection fraction (EF) under 35% on optimal medical therapy.[27] This trial was an open-label comparison of empiric amiodarone and standard therapy for HF. With a primary endpoint of mortality, the trial, after a mean follow-up of 13 months, demonstrated a significant reduction in all-cause mortality, 41.4% versus 33.5% ($P$=0.024), respectively. No significant reduction was found when the data were analyzed by mode of death, HF or SCD. The secondary outcome was death or hospital admission for congestive heart failure (CHF). In this trial, amiodarone was associated with a significant reduction of the secondary endpoint, from 58.2% to 48.5% ($P$=0.0024).

The second major trial investigating the use of amiodarone in HF patients to reduce mortality was a US Veterans Affairs-sponsored study known as the CHF Survival Trial of Antiarrhythmic Therapy (CHF-STAT).[28] CHF-STAT was a placebo-controlled trial of amiodarone in patients with HF and ambient ventricular arrhythmia. In this trial, amiodarone demonstrated no mortality benefit for the total population, but a subgroup analysis identified a trend suggesting that the non-ischemic cardiomyopathy group might benefit from amiodarone therapy. The CAD subgroup (70% of the enrollees) showed no benefit.

Neither CHF-STAT nor GESICA allowed a definitive conclusion regarding amiodarone as a primary prevention strategy to decrease mortality in patients with HF. Ultimately, this was addressed in the SCD Heart Failure Trial (SCD-HeFT).[29]

### The implantable defibrillator and SCD prevention

Strategies to prevent SCD in high-risk patients with CAD and HF in the past two decades have primarily focused on the use of the implantable defibrillator. As the technology improved to transvenous devices with small generator volume allowing the placement of the ICD in the prepectoral space, the widespread use of the ICD became a viable option. Given the dismal survival rates worldwide of victims of

SCD, strategies aimed at primary prevention were developed. Identifying high-risk patients most likely to benefit from ICD therapy proved to be difficult, due in part to the heterogeneity of the HF population, lack of understanding of the mechanisms involved, severity of HF, and etiology of HF. The mortality data from the HF trials of medical therapy[23,30] did demonstrate consistently two facts. First, with increasing severity of HF, the risk of sudden death increases. Second, as the severity of HF increases, the percentage of deaths accounted for by SCD diminishes. These findings support the focus of ICD therapy on those with moderate symptoms of HF.

## ICD therapy in high-risk CAD patients

Initial trials examining the role of ICD therapy in primary prevention patients focused on high-risk CAD patients. These trials include CABG-Patch, MADIT, MUSTT and MADIT II, the last of which is the most relevant to current practice.[31–34]

The CABG-Patch trial used predominantly epicardial devices, and randomized only patients already deemed to require surgical coronary revascularization, the likely major risk reduction intervention in these patients.[31] This intervention and the use of a higher-risk epicardial leads system probably explain the absence of a survival benefit from the ICD in this trial.

The early MADIT identified a very select group of patients with high-risk CAD and persistent electrophysiologic (EP) inducibility, and randomized 196 patients to an ICD or to 'conventional' medical therapy. Amiodarone, beta-blockers, or any other antiarrhythmic therapy did not influence the observed outcome. A dramatic reduction in total mortality (56%) was seen in the ICD arm.[32] This was viewed with both skepticism (because of lack of broad applicability and low use of beta-blocker therapy) and enthusiasm (for its dramatically reduced mortality) and supported the implementation of the larger MADIT II trial.

The MUSTT trial was designed to test the hypothesis that EP guided antiarrhythmic treatment would reduce the risk of SD in high risk CAD patients and reduced left ventricular function (EF $<40\%$).[33] However, many patients' inducible tachycardia could not be suppressed by medication. The 5-year rates of cardiac arrest or death from arrhythmia were 9% in patients receiving EP-guided ICD implantation versus 37% in those who did not receive an ICD ($P<0.001$), a relative risk reduction of $>70\%$. A significant survival advantage was noted in the patients randomized to a strategy of EP testing, however, was entirely due to the use of the ICD in that arm of the trial. These results have been used to support the ICD in high-risk CAD patients with EF of $<40\%$ and inducible VT/VF during EP studies.

The MADIT II trial was designed to have broader applicability by eliminating the requirement for EP testing.[34] To increase the risk of the study population, the entry EF requirement was decreased from 35% (MADIT) to 30%. Patients could be in NYHA class I, II or III. The trial evaluated 1232 patients with prior MI greater than one month prior to randomization and with left ventricular ejection fraction (LVEF) of $\leq 30\%$. Patients were randomized in a 3:2 ratio to ICD ($n=742$) or conventional medical therapy ($n=490$), including beta-blockers, ACE inhibitors, and lipid-lowering therapy. The primary endpoint was all-cause mortality.

Baseline characteristics were well matched in the treatment groups. Most patients had experienced their MI greater than 6 months before enrollment. Most patients were taking ACE inhibitors, diuretics, and beta-blockers. Over a mean follow-up of 20 months, all cause mortality rates were 19.8% and 14.2% in the drug and ICD treatment groups, respectively, accounting for a 31% relative risk reduction

($P=0.016$).[34] The benefit of the ICD was subsequently shown to increase as the time interval between an individual's prior MI and enrollment in the trial.[35]

The results of the MADIT II trial dramatically increased the number of potential ICD candidates. In an attempt to identify those patients most likely to benefit, the US Center for Medicare and Medicaid Services (CMS) conducted a post-hoc analysis of the data. The observation that the benefit appeared to be greater in those individuals with a QRS width of >120 ms resulted in limiting reimbursement to patients meeting the QRS width requirement.

## ICD therapy in HF

The two trials that specifically addressed a population of patients with moderate HF were the SCD-HeFT and the Prophylactic Defibrillator Implantation in Patients with Nonischemic Dilated Cardiomyopathy Treatment Evaluation (DEFINITE)[29,36] trials. Only SCD-HeFT included patients with both ischemic and nonischemic causes of cardiomyopathy and an amiodarone/placebo arm.

DEFINITE examined only patients with nonischemic cardiomyopathy and did not include an antiarrhythmic drug therapy arm.[36] The 458 patients with LVEF of <36%, were randomized to control (good background HF medical therapy) or single lead ICD therapy. The primary endpoint was total mortality. At an average follow-up of 29 months, the trial did not demonstrate a statistically significant reduction in all-cause mortality.

The SCD-HeFT trial is the most recent and largest randomized, controlled trial assessing ICD therapy for either primary or secondary prevention and has the longest follow-up of any ICD trial to date (median follow-up of 45.5 months). SCD-HeFT is a multicenter, prospective, randomized trial that compared ICD to placebo-controlled amiodarone in patients with class II or III HF with either an ischemic or nonischemic cause of cardiomyopathy. The primary endpoint of the trial was total mortality, with secondary endpoints that included cardiac and arrhythmic mortality. The enrollment criteria were designed to have ultimately broad applicability to the practicing clinician, and required only that participants have an EF of ≤35%, and be class II or III HF patients who had been stabilized on vasodilator (ACE or ARB) therapy for at least 2 weeks. All patients underwent a 12-lead ECG, a 6-min walk test, and a Holter monitor for the purpose of subsequent substudies. Exclusion criteria included history of cardiac arrest, unexplained syncope within 5 years, indication for pacemaker implantation, current amiodarone, contraindications to amiodarone, or requirement for antiarrhythmic drug usage other than calcium-channel blockers, beta-blockers, or digoxin. The ICD used was a single-lead device programmed conservatively to include only a single zone of shock-only therapy and back-up single-chamber (VVI) pacing at 50 bpm (hysteresis of 34 bpm).

The 2521 patients were randomized in equal proportions to one of the three treatment arms. There were 847 patients randomized to placebo plus conventional HF therapy, 845 randomized to blinded amiodarone plus conventional HF therapy, and 829 randomized to the ICD plus conventional HF therapy. The enrollment scheme included prestratification based upon HF class and cause of cardiomyopathy.

Patients with a nonischemic cause of HF comprised 48% of the patients; ischemic cause of HF accounted for the other 52% of patients. Class II HF patients comprised 70% of the population, while class III patients represented the other 30%. Class I and IV patients were excluded from enrollment. Other notable clinical characteristics include the fact that men represented 77% of the study population, the median age was 59.5 years, and median LVEF was 24%. Excellent background HF therapy was achieved in this trial (96% were on ACE or ARB, and 69% on beta-blocker therapy at enrollment), especially considering that the results of the major trials demonstrating a survival benefit from beta-blocker therapy were not completed when this trial began. By the end of the trial, 78% of the patients were on beta-blocker therapy.

Two of the unique features of the SCD-HeFT study design were the use of only a single-lead ICD and programming that excluded antitachycardia pacing. Although the results of the later dual-chamber and VVI implantable defibrillator (DAVID) trial showing higher mortality associated with ICD dual-chamber pacing had not yet been published, it was a specific strategy of the SCD-HeFT investigators to control ICD usage and avoid the bias that would otherwise occur if the choice of programming and device technology was left to the investigators' discretion.[32,34,37]

The primary results of the trial showed no overall mortality benefit for amiodarone therapy compared to placebo (HR=1.06, 97.5% CI: 0.86–1.30), while single-lead ICD therapy reduced mortality by 23% (HR=0.77, 97.5% CI: 0.62–0.96, $P$=0.007) compared to placebo (Figure 6.2). The benefit of the ICD was in addition to excellent background HF medical therapy, which, alone, resulted in a placebo mortality rate of only 7.2% per year.

Subgroup analysis demonstrated that the benefit of the ICD appeared limited to the patients with NYHA class II HF (HR=0.54, 97.5% CI: 0.40–0.74, $P<0.001$), while class III patients appeared not to benefit (HR=1.16, 97.5% CI: 0.84–1.61, $P$=0.30) (Figure 6.2). Moreover, class III patients treated with amiodarone appeared to have an increased risk of death (HR=1.44), while class II patients showed no difference between amiodarone therapy and placebo (HR=0.85). The lack of benefit associated with amiodarone was the same regardless of the cause of cardiomyopathy.

The results of the SCD-HeFT trial broadened the US Medicare reimbursement for ICD implantation to include both high-risk patients with ischemic heart disease (EF ≤35%) and those with nonischemic HF (EF≤35%). Importantly, the earlier restriction to include only those patients with a QRS>120 ms was eliminated after a substudy analysis of SCD-HeFT demonstrated no significant interaction of QRS width and the mortality reduction observed with the ICD.[38]

### Insights from primary prevention ICD trials

SCD-HeFT demonstrated no mortality reduction with amiodarone therapy compared to placebo in this population, effectively settling the question of amiodarone's role in primary prevention of SCD. Subgroup analysis shows a consistent lack of benefit in NYHA class II patients but suggested that a possible harmful effect in NYHA class III patients. The causes of this excess mortality are not immediately obvious, in that significant amiodarone side effects were low,[29] and further analysis of the data is required. There is a practical concern, however, in that amiodarone is frequently used, and it is often the only antiarrhythmic drug choice to treat atrial fibrillation, a commonly occurring rhythm disturbance in HF patients and a significant cause of inappropriate ICD therapy.

The finding that patients with NYHA class II HF appeared to benefit the most from ICD therapy and that class III patients appeared to derive no survival advantage may not have been an anticipated outcome of the trial. There are two important aspects of this class difference. First, the patients with healthier hearts (class II) may actually be more likely to be overlooked for ICD therapy. This is because they seem to be doing well on routine clinic visits, are less often seen in the outpatient setting,

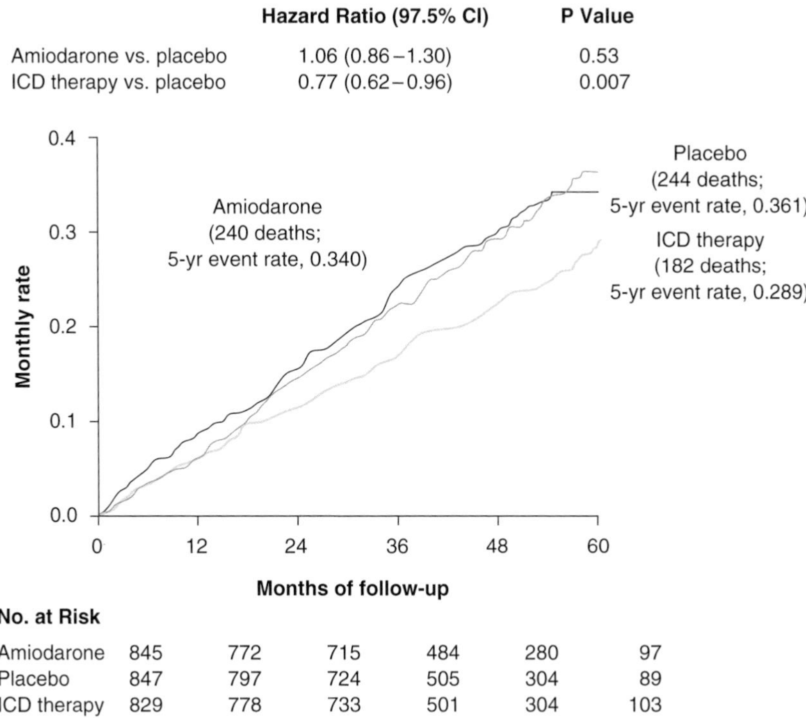


**Figure 6.1** Kaplan–Meier estimates of death from any cause. CI: confidence interval.

and are less likely to be followed by the specialist with cardiology/HF expertise; yet, these are the patients who are generally leading productive and functional lives and thus, have the most to gain from ICD therapy. Second, contrary to earlier presumptions, patients with NYHA class III HF may not benefit from ICD therapy because death from advanced HF outweighs the benefit of appropriate ICD therapy for life-threatening ventricular arrhythmia. Comparative data on class III patients are limited. A subgroup analysis of class III patients from the DEFINITE trial (96 patients), demonstrating a survival advantage of the ICD over background HF therapy in the 96 NYHA class III patients.[36] These data have been used to support the use of ICD therapy in class III patients. In a post-hoc analysis of the MADIT II data,[39] a small and statistically insignificant survival benefit in favor of the ICD was seen in the class III patients ($P$=0.216). Although these data might preclude conclusions being drawn regarding the benefit or lack thereof of the ICD in class III patients, the SCD-HeFT results represent 760 randomized patients, the largest analysis of class III patients treated with an ICD in any clinical trial of ICD primary prevention therapy. One possible explanation of the conflicting results with class III patients might be the subjective vagaries inherent in ascribing the NYHA class II versus class III label to an individual patient. However, in a separate analysis comparing the benefit of the ICD with placebo, stratifying the SCD-HeFT patients according to 6-min walk ability showed consistent results. That is, the patients with the worse 6-min walk (<950 feet) did not have a reduction in mortality with ICD

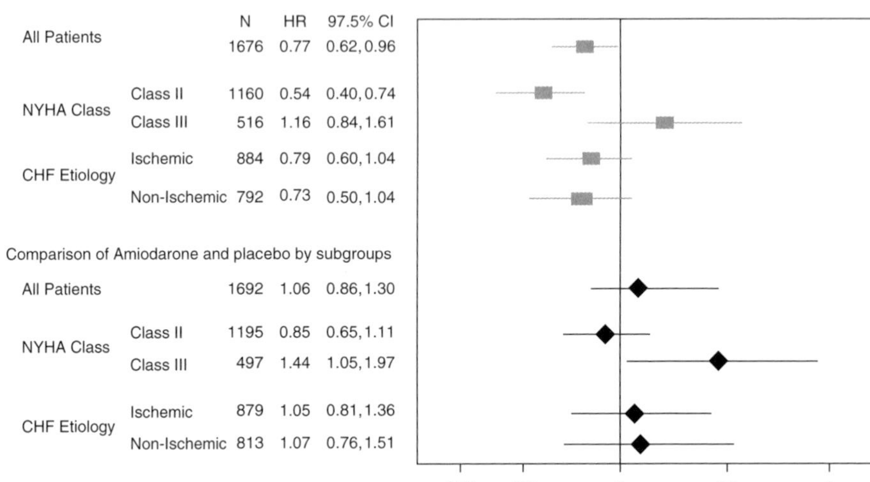


**Figure 6.2** Kaplan–Meier estimates of death from any cause for the prespecified subgroups of NYHA class II and class III. CI: confidence interval.

therapy compared to those patients with ≥950 feet.[40] These are remarkably consistent results and certainly, bring into question the benefit of the ICD in class III patients. Whether or not these findings are simply a 'quirk' of clinical trial statistics and post-hoc subgroup analysis is unknown and would require further studies designed to evaluate the role of the ICD in class III patients. Short of such data being available, it is reasonable to recommend that ICDs should be implanted in NYHA Class II and III HF patients with EF ≤35% with either an ischemic or non-ischemic cause of the HF.

The only other data on class III (and class IV) patients are limited to those with a wide QRS and are available only from industry-sponsored studies of cardiac resynchronization therapy (CRT). The Comparison of Medical Therapy, Pacing, and Defibrillation in HF (COMPANION) trial randomized 1520 patients in unequal proportions to CRT with an ICD, to a CRT pacemaker alone, or to open-label standard drug therapy for HF.[41] The trial demonstrated that CRT-ICD and CRT-pacemaker were equally effective at reducing the combined endpoint of all-cause mortality and rehospitalization for any cause compared to control patients. The secondary endpoint of all-cause mortality was significantly reduced by the CRT-ICD ($P=0.0059$), but not the CRT-pacemaker, leaving open the possibility that the defibrillator alone was responsible for the reduction in deaths. In contrast to this outcome, the Cardiac Resynchronization-HF (CARE-HF) randomized 813 patients to a CRT-pacemaker (no ICD) compared to standard open-label drug therapy for CHF.[42] CRT significantly decreased the primary endpoint of the trial, which was all-cause mortality plus unplanned rehospitalization for a major cardiovascular event. CRT-only therapy decreased the secondary endpoint of mortality by 36% (HR=0.64; 95% CI: 0.48–0.85, $P<0.002$). The results of these two trials leave us with an unclear understanding of the relative benefit of CRT pacemaker alone compared to CRT-ICD in patients with moderate to severe HF and a wide QRS, in that both appear to be associated with reduction in mortality.

### ICD therapy in the acute post-MI patient

One final trial of ICD therapy in high-risk patients deserves comment. The Defibrillator in Acute Myocardial Infarction Trial (DINAMIT) was a clinical trial in which patients with recent MI (6-40 days), autonomic dysfunction with reduced heart rate variability, and LVEF of ≤35% were randomized to either ICD (332 patients) or optimal medical therapy (342 patients). Over 30 months, there was no significant difference detected in the primary outcome, death from any cause ($P=0.66$). As expected, ICD therapy was associated with significantly fewer arrhythmic deaths than in the medical therapy group ($P=0.009$); however, the number of nonarrhythmic deaths was also significantly higher in the ICD group ($P=0.02$).[43]

One explanation might be the relatively low mortality in the control group, where use of background medical therapy was robust (beta-blockers in 87%, ACE inhibitors in 94%, and lipid-lowering agents in >76%). The use of statin therapy in acute MI has received recent attention, as it appears to improve short-term outcomes following acute MI via mechanisms that have not yet been fully understood.[44,45]

An additional explanation may be that the ICD itself was responsible for excess mortality despite appropriate ICD detection and shock delivery for appropriate VT or VF. This group of patients had very high mortality, and the result of ICD therapy may have been to convert mode of death from arrhythmic death to pump failure death. Given the findings of this study, there seems to be little justification for routine implantation of an ICD in the first 4 weeks after MI. A reasonable alternative to ICD implantation in these patients would be to embrace widespread automated external defibrillators or wearable defibrillators for these individuals.

## CONCLUSION

Medical therapy alone has improved survival in HF patients dramatically over the past 20 years. Despite the many advances, sudden death remains an important clinical challenge in these patients. Numerous attempts have been made to discern discriminators for survival, although measures of left ventricular function either by EF or HF classification, remains the most predictive clinical feature with which to assess a patient's risk of SCD. Data from the large clinical ICD trials, targeting specifically moderate-risk HF patients, have without question demonstrated a survival benefit associated with ICD therapy in high-risk patients, both with and without CAD. Given that the economic implications of widespread use of ICD therapy, particularly when CRT is included, are substantial, further trials would be required to identify the relative benefit of ICD, CRT or combined ICD-CRT in high risk subgroups.

## REFERENCES


1. Zipes DP, Wellens HJ. Sudden cardiac death. Circulation 1998; 98: 2334–51.
2. American Heart Association. 2005 Heart and Stroke Statistical Update. Dallas, TX: American Heart Association, 2005.
3. De Vreede-Swageemakers JJ, Gorgels AP, Dubois-Arbouw WI et al. Out-of-hospital cardiac arrest in the 1990's: a population-based study in the Maastricht area on incidence, characteristics and survival. J Am Coll Cardiol 1997; 30: 1500–5.
4. Myerburg RJ, Interian AJ, Mitrani RM et al. Frequency of sudden cardiac death and profiles of risk. Am J Cardiol 1997; 80: 10F–19F.
5. Myerburg RJ, Kessler KM, Castellanos A. Sudden cardiac death. Structure, function, and time-dependence of risk. Circulation 1992; 85: I2–I10.
6. Becker LB, Ostrander MP, Barrett J et al. Outcome of CPR in a large metropolitan area: where are the survivors? Ann Emerg Med 1991; 20: 355–61.

7. Lombardi G, Gallagher J, Gennis P. Outcome of out-of-hospital cardiac arrest in New York City: the pre-hospital arrest survival evaluation study. JAMA 1994; 271: 678–83.
8. Eisenberg MS, Horwood BT, Cummins RO et al. Cardiac arrest and resuscitation: a tale of 29 cities. Ann Emerg Med 1990; 19: 179–86.
9. Davies M, Hobbs F, Davis R et al. Prevalence of left-ventricular systolic dysfunction and heart failure in the Echocardiographic Heart of England Screening study: a population based study. Lancet 2001; 358: 439–44.
10. Levy D, Kenchaiah S, Larson MG et al. Long-term trends in the incidence of and survival with heart failure. N Engl J Med 2002; 347: 1397–402.
11. Rose EA, Gelijns AC, Moskowitz AJ et al. Long-term mechanical left ventricular assistance for end-stage heart failure. N Engl J Med 2001; 345: 1435–43.
12. MERIT-HF Study Group. Effect of metoprolol CR/XL in chronic heart failure: Metoprolol CR/XL Randomised Intervention Trial in Congestive Heart Failure (MERIT-HF). Lancet 1999; 353: 2001–7.
13. Ellison KE, Stevenson WG, Sweeney MO et al. Management of arrhythmias in heart failure. Congest Heart Fail 2003; 9: 91–9.
14. Saxon LA, De Marco T, Prystowsky EN et al. Resynchronization therapy for heart failure. Educational Content From the Heart Rhythm Society. www.hrsonline.org/uploadDocs/CRT_12_3.pdf (accessed 22 July, 2005).
15. Xiao HB, Lee CH, Gibson DG: Effect of left bundle branch block on diastolic function in dilated cardiomyopathy. Br Heart J 1991; 66: 443–7.
16. CIBIS-II Investigators and Committees: the Cardiac Insufficiency Bisoprolol Study II (CIBIS II): a randomized trial. Lancet 1999; 353: 9–13.
17. Packer M, Bristow M, Cohn J et al. The effect of carvedilol on mortality and morbidity in patients with chronic heart failure. N Engl J Med 1996; 334: 1349–55.
18. Poole-Wilson PA, Swedberg K, Cleland JGF et al. Comparison of carvedilol and metoprolol on clinical outcomes in patients with chronic heart failure in the carvedilol or metoprolol European trial (COMET): randomized controlled trial. Lancet 2003; 362: 7–13.
19. Packer M, Coats AJ, Fowler M et al. Effect of carvedilol on survival in severe chronic heart failure. N Engl J Med 2001; 344: 1659–67.
20. The CAPRICORN investigators. Effect of carvedilol on outcome after myocardial infarction in patients with left-ventricular dysfunction: the CAPRICORN randomized trial. Lancet 2001; 357: 1385–90.
21. Packer M, Poole-Wilson PA, Armstrong PW et al. Comparative effects of low and high doses of the angiotensin converting enzyme inhibitor, lisinopril, on morbidity and mortality in chronic heart failure. ATLAS study group. Circulation 1999; 100: 2312–8.
22. Poole-Wilson PA, Uretsky BF, Thygesen K et al. Mode of death in heart failure: findings from the ATLAS trial. Heart 2003; 89: 42–8.
23. MERIT-HF investigators, Effect of metoprolol CR/XL in chronic heart failure: Metoprolol CR/XL Randomised Intervention Trial in Congestive Heart Failure (MERIT-HF). Lancet 1999; 353: 2001–7.
24. Poole-Wilson PA, Swedberg K, Cleland JG et al. Comparison of carvedilol and metoprolol on clinical outcomes in patients with chronic heart failure in the carvedilol or metoprolol European trial (COMET): randomized controlled trial. Lancet 2004; 362: 7–13.
25. Willenheimer R, van Veldhuisen DJ, Silke B et al. Effect on survival and hospitalization of initiating treatment for chronic heart failure with bisoprolol followed by enalapril, as compared with the opposite sequence. Results of the randomized cardiac insufficiency bisoprolol study (CIBIS) III. Circulation 2005; 112(16): 2426–35.
26. Sliwa K, Norton GR, Kone N et al. Impact of initiating carvedilol before angiotensin-converting enzyme inhibitor therapy on cardiac function in newly diagnosed heart failure. J Am Coll Cardiol 2004; 44: 1825–30.
27. Wilber DJ, Zareba W, Hall WJ et al. Time dependence of mortality risk and defibrillator benefit after myocardial infarction. Circulation 2004; 109(9): 1082–4.

28. Singh SN, Fletcher RD, Fisher SG et al for the Survival Trial of Antiarrhythmic Therapy in Congestive Heart Failure: amiodarone in patients with congestive heart failure and asymptomatic ventricular arrhythmia. N Engl J Med 1995; 333: 77–82.
29. Bardy GH, Lee KL, Mark DB et al. Amiodarone or an implantable cardioverter-defibrillator for congestive heart failure. N Engl J Med 2005; 352: 225–37.
30. Goldman S, Johnson G, Cohn JN. Mechanisms of death in heart failure: the vasodilator-heart failure trials. the V-HeFT VA Cooperative Studies Group. Circulation 1993; 87: V124–V131.
31. Bigger JT Jr. Prophylactic use of implanted cardiac defibrillators in patients at high risk for ventricular arrhythmias after coronary artery bypass graft surgery. N Engl J Med 1997; 337: 1569–75.
32. Moss AJ Hall WJ, Cannom DS et al. Improved survival with an implantable defibrillator in patients with coronary disease at high risk for ventricular arrhythmia. Multicenter Automatic Defibrillator Implantation Trial Investigators. N Engl J Med 1996; 335: 133–40.
33. Buxton AE, Lee KL, Fisher JD et al. A randomized study of the prevention of sudden death in patients with coronary artery disease. Multicenter Unsustained Tachycardia Trial Investigators. N Engl J Med 1999; 341: 1882–90.
34. Moss AJ, Zareba W, Hall WJ et al, Multicenter Automatic Defibrillator Implantation Trial II Investigators: prophylactic implantation of a defibrillator in patients with myocardial infarction and reduced ejection fraction. N Engl J Med 2002; 346: 877–83.
35. Wilber DJ, Zareba W, Hall WF, Brown M, Moss AJ: Time-dependence of mortality risk and defibrillator benefit following myocardial infarction: lessons from the Multicenter Automatic Defibrillator Implantation Trial II. PACE 2003; 26(part 2): 961 (Abstract 130).
36. Kadish A, Dyer A, Daubert JP: Prophylactic defibrillator implantation in patients with nonischemic dilated cardiomyopathy. N Engl J Med 2004; 350: 2151–8.
37. Wilkoff BL, Cook JR, Epstein AE et al. Dual-chamber pacing or ventricular backup pacing in patients with an implantable defibrillator. The dual chamber and VVI implantable defibrillator (DAVID) trial. JAMA 2002; 288: 3115–23.
38. Poole JE, Anderson J, Johnson GW et al. Baseline ECG data and outcome in the Sudden Cardiac Death-Heart Failure Trial. NASPE Heart Rhythm Society, May 2004, San Diego CA.
39. Zareba W, Piotrowicz K, McNitt S, Moss AJ for the MADIT II Investigators. Implantable cardioverter-defibrillator efficacy in patients with heart failure and left ventricular dysfunction (from the MADIT II population). Am J Cardiol 2005; 95: 1487–91.
40. Fishbein DP, Walsh MN, Poole JE et al. Baseline 6 minute walk distance in the Sudden Cardiac Death Heart Failure Trial. American Heart Association Scientific Sessions 2004, 7–10, November 2004, New Orleans, LA.
41. Bristow MR, Saxon LA, Boehmer J et al, for the Comparison of Medical Therapy, Pacing, and Defibrillation in Heart Failure (COMPANION) Investigators. Cardiac-resynchronization therapy with or without an implantable defibrillator in advanced chronic heart failure. N Engl J Med 2004; 350: 2140–50.
42. Cleland JG, Tavazzi L, Daubert JC et al, for the CARE HF Investigators. The Cardiac Resynchronization Heart Failure Study (CARE-HF): a randomized study of the effects of optimal pharmacological therapy alone or combined with cardiac resynchronization in patients with advanced heart failure and cardiac dyssynchrony. N Engl J Med 2005A; 352: 1539–49.
43. Hohnloser SH, Kuck KH, Dorian P et al, on behalf of the DINAMIT Investigators. Prophylactic use of an implantable cardioverter-defibrillator after acute myocardial infarction.
N Engl J Med 2004; 351: 2481–8.
44. Stenestrand U, Wallentin L, for the Swedish Register of Cardiac Intensive Care (RIKS-HIA). Early statin treatment following acute myocardial infarction and 1-year survival. JAMA 2001; 285: 430–6.
45. Chan AW, Bhatt DL, Chew, DP et al. Early and sustained survival benefit associated with statin therapy at the time of percutaneous coronary intervention. Circulation 2002; 105: 691.

# 7

# Early defibrillation program: the future of public defibrillation

Alessandro Capucci and Daniela Aschieri

Approaches to the prevention of sudden cardiac death (SCD) include strategies designed to attack the problem from multiple perspectives: primary prevention of the underlying diseases, prophylactic treatment of high-risk individuals with already identified diseases, and responses to cardiac arrest victims in the community. The latter strategy began with conventional fire department-based emergency rescue systems (EMS) that originated in the early 1970s in the USA.

Newer early intervention strategies include a variety of methods, including ambulance- and police-based automatic external defibrillators (AEDs), deployment of AEDs in crowd settings with designated rescuers, and more general public access sites. The value of conventional EMS systems lies in their ability to provide advanced life support as part of a dual-response system. The new technology allows defibrillation to be performed by a wide variety of individuals with diverse backgrounds and training.

## CHEST COMPRESSION AND VENTILATION IN THE CHAIN OF SURVIVAL

The optimal strategy to treat sudden out-of-hospital cardiac arrest should be primary prevention of the event. However, this approach is currently limited by our inability to identify prospectively the majority of potential SCD victims. We also do not yet have a safe, effective, and inexpensive preventive drug or device for the majority of potential victims. Moreover, an acute myocardial infarction may start as a sudden phenomenon in a coronary vassel without any previous significant stenosis and therefore may hardly be foreseen.

The American Heart Association has developed a *chain of survival* strategy that is designed to optimize a patient's chance for survival of out-of-hospital cardiac arrest.[1] There are four links in the chain: 1) early access; 2) early cardiopulmonary resuscitation (CPR); 3) early defibrillation; and 4) early advanced cardiac life support (ACLS). *Early access* means that citizens have been trained to recognize out-of-hospital cardiac arrest quickly and that a system of communications and emergency medical dispatch is in place to send trained emergency medical personnel and equipment quickly to the scene. *Early CPR* by bystanders provides ventilation and circulation support, buying precious minutes for emergency medical teams (or someone else) to arrive with a defibrillator to perform *defibrillation* and other *advanced life support* equipment.

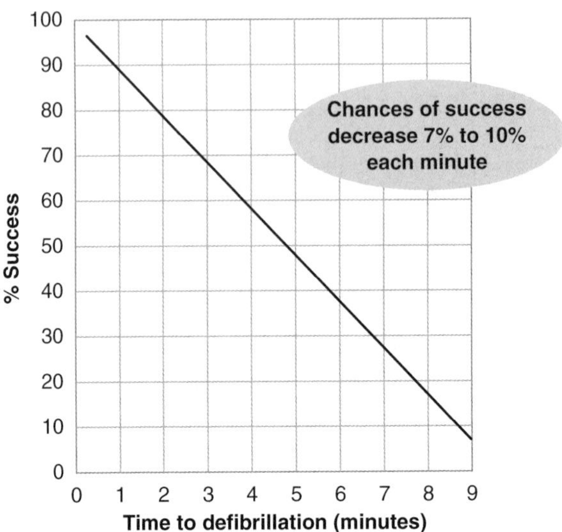


**Figure 7.1** Time dependence of survival after cardiac arrest.

Only a few communities have developed a strong chain of survival that yields significantly improved survival from out-of-hospital cardiac arrest. For more than 30 years, CPR has been refined by leading researchers and performed by many rescuers. Without doubt, the procedure helps to save many lives. The likelihood of survival is estimated to decrease by 5–10%/min after the onset of cardiac arrest (Figure 7.1), although there is evidence that this is not a linear function. Rapid implementation of CPR has emerged as the highest priority. For example in Seattle, Washington, 27% of patients with witnessed out-of-hospital cardiac arrest survived when bystanders performed CPR; only 13% survived without bystander CPR.[2]

This was the incentive for Eisenberg et al[3] to initiate a program of bystander-initiated CPR to train the general public.

However, CPR alone prolongs life, rather than saves it. In rural areas where emergency vehicles are nonexistent or too far away, survival rates are extremely low even when CPR is applied. Similarly, in many urban areas, such as Chicago, a very low survival rate was recorded (overall 1.7% survival rate from out-of-hospital cardiac arrest) in 1987[4] with the traditional medical service system. Similar results were demonstrated in 1991 in New York City, where only 1.4% of victims survived,[5] average response times for ambulance services with defibrillators were greater than 10–12 min. These poor outcomes reflect the short time within which CPR is effective. In fact, CPR simply buys the victim a few more minutes of precious time waiting for defibrillation, since CPR can artificially circulate only up to 30% of the body's original blood volume. CPR is useful when defibrillation comes soon, but only modest results are obtained when defibrillation time is longer than 10 min.

## New defibrillators

Recent advances in AED technology and design have resulted in marked simplification of AED operation, improvements in accuracy and effectiveness, and reductions

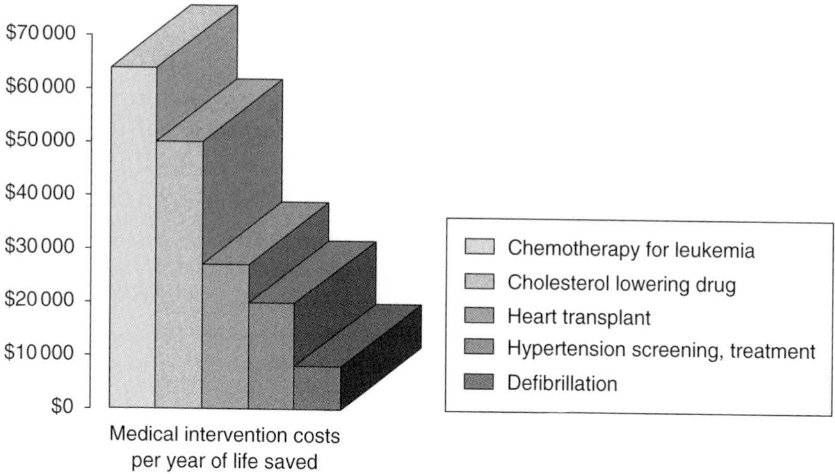


**Figure 7.2** Cost-effectiveness of AED use in comparison with other commonly used treatment is favorable.

in cost. Use of AEDs by first responders and laypersons has reduced the time to defibrillation and improved survival rates from sudden cardiac arrest in several communities. Initial studies of the cost-effectiveness of AED use in comparison with other commonly used treatments are favorable. The cost of first-responder AED programs over 5 years was $4400–$8000 per year of life saved. This cost compares favorably with costs of other medical interventions (Figure 7.2). AEDs today require the placement of pads at the right sternal border and at the cardiac apex. These electrodes serve to monitor and to defibrillate. By means of a vocal message, AEDs can also inform the user when lead contact is poor, when the machine is preparing to defibrillate, when to check for a pulse, when a nonshockable rhythm is present, or when motion is detected.

### Full automatic versus semiautomatic

Fully automatic AEDs shock at preprogrammed levels once ventricular fibrillation (VF) or ventricular tachycardia is sensed. Electrodes are placed in position, and the AED is turned on after confirming that the patient is in cardiac arrest. The only way to prevent firing once the machine is committed to discharge is by turning 'off' the AED. Semiautomatic models inform the user when VF or ventricular tachycardia is sensed, and then advise defibrillation. The operator must not press a button to deliver the shock. The user can discharge the unit whenever necessary, even if this is not advised so in the manual version. With many of the models, the operator can override the AED.

### Rhythm analysis

Early AEDs were designed to respond primarily to a heart rate greater than 150 electrical complexes per min and an electrocardiographic wave (QRS) amplitude greater than 0.15 ms. Presently, the ECG rhythm is analyzed via a combination of several

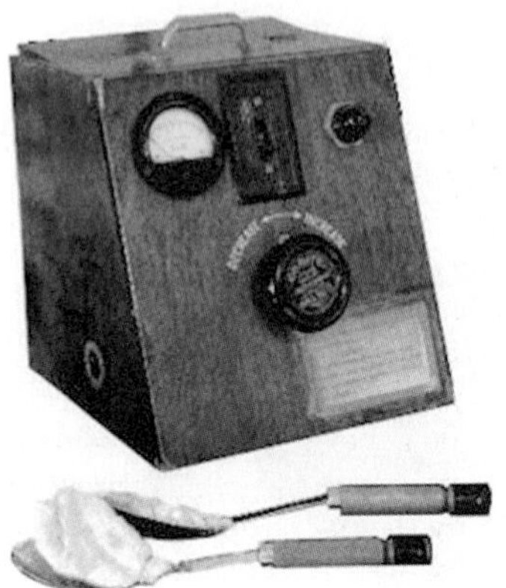

**Year 1947**
**Claude Beck, defibrillator**

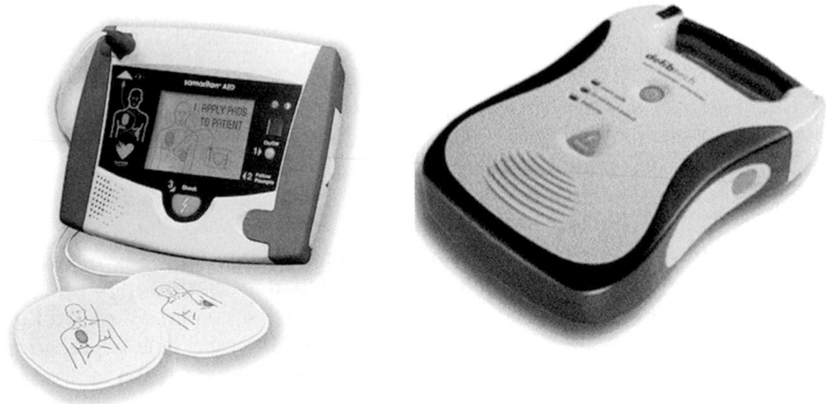


**Year 2004**
**Samaritan Defibrillator for home use**

**Figure 7.3** Evolution of defibrillators.

methods. In addition to rate and amplitude criteria, the QRS is analyzed as to its slope, morphology, power spectrum density, and time away from the isoelectric baseline for preset levels defined as abnormal. Checks are made at 2–4-s intervals. In general, if abnormal complexes are detected for more than double the frequency of any other QRS for three consecutive checks, the AED will be primed to deliver a shock. Fine VF presents the greatest detection challenge. A trade-off exists between setting the amplitude criterion low enough to detect fine fibrillation, yet high enough to avoid shocking asystole or artifact. The sensitivity of detecting VF by AEDs has been reported as 76–96%. Specificity (correctly identifying non-VF rhythms) is reported to be nearly 100%.

**Early defibrillation: the perspectives**

We can identify five levels of potential AED users:

1. traditional responders (trained persons who have a duty to respond to medical emergencies, e.g., EMS personnel)
2. first responders (trained individuals with a duty to respond to emergencies and likely to react to a medical emergency, e.g., police, firefighters)
3. volunteer nonmedical responders (trained individuals without a duty to respond to medical emergencies as their primary job description who desire to be trained to assume that duty; e.g., store managers, office clerks, building superintendents, and other members of the general public)
4. untrained members of the lay public (e.g., passersby)
5. family members of individuals known to be at risk of out-of-hospital cardiac arrest.

There are four possible strategies to organize an early defibrillation program:

1. defibrillation in ambulances (medical technicians or ambulance volunteers)
2. defibrillation by first responders such as police officers and firefighters (early defibrillation), creating a two-tier response system (ambulance and first responders)
3. defibrillation in public places with lay people trained in their use
4. home defibrillation.

*1) Rapid defibrillation: AEDs in the ambulance*

The ambulance system may provide rapid defibrillation to out-of-hospital cardiac arrest victims throughout the ambulance staff (nonmedical or medical personnel). The first defibrillators were large and heavy (Figure 7.3 top), making them unsuitable for transport. In 1962, Bernard Lown developed a direct-current defibrillator, which decreased the need for a large-capacity transformer and therefore allowed the manufacture of substantially lighter and smaller defibrillators. The greatest initial impact was for use on patients with acute myocardial infarction, thus beginning the era of mobile coronary care. Defibrillation allowed an impressive decrease in 48-h mortality among patients with ischemic heart disease; witnessed cardiac arrest due to VF was almost immediately reversed with prompt defibrillation.

In 1967, in Belfast, Dr Frank Pantridge was the first to show that victims of SCD could be successfully resuscitated outside the hospital. As the project continued and greater numbers of patients became available for study, the Belfast investigators found that the time it took from onset of cardiac arrest to the first defibrillation attempt was the single most significant factor in determining a successful resuscitation.

The innovative Belfast program was of primary importance for the development of ALS systems throughout Europe and the USA. But despite this experience, over the past three decades, the EMS has had several difficulties in optimizing sudden cardiac arrest survival rates. Even now, very few ambulances carry a defibrillator on board. The medical staff are often required to perform defibrillation even in the presence of paramedic personnel. A recent meta-analysis of 10 studies demonstrated a 9.2% absolute increase in survival when basic emergency medical technicians (EMTs) used AEDs in the field.[6]

*2) Early defibrillation by first responders*

The term 'early defibrillation' suggests defibrillation within 5 min after collapse. Even if this is seldom achieved by the ambulance system, recent studies have clearly demonstrated that early defibrillation may be done with AEDs used by trained public-safety personnel ('first responders'), so-called nontraditional rescuers.

AEDs can automatically detect and treat VF so making it possible for public-safety personnel (EMT basics, police, and firefighters) to defibrillate safely. Clinical trials of AEDs used by EMT basics have shown, with few exceptions, that this technology is safe and saves lives. These devices defibrillate the heart with a high degree of sensitivity and specificity. However, about 24% of EMS in the USA still lack defibrillation capability.[7] In Europe, there is no unique emergency system, and no unique data base exists.

*Preliminary studies on early defibrillation.* Studies on first-responder systems of early defibrillation clearly demonstrated that first responders can safely and effectively defibrillate in the field[8–20] (Table 7.1). The initial results have not been as striking, although they are over a decade old and were conducted at a time when the technology was much less sophisticated, and devices were more difficult to use. In Seattle, Weaver et al[13] compared the results of initial treatment with this device by firefighters who arrived first on the scene, as compared with the results of standard defibrillation administered by paramedics who arrived slightly later than the firefighters. Of 276 patients who were initially treated by firefighters with the AED, 84 (30%) survived to hospital discharge as compared with 44 (19%) of 228 patients when firefighters delivered only basic CPR, and the first defibrillation was performed after the arrival of the paramedic team. The main factors influencing survival after VF were witnessed collapse, younger age, the presence of 'coarse' (higher-amplitude) fibrillation, a shorter response time for paramedics, and initial treatment by firefighters with an AED. Chadda and Kammerer[21] trained a group of responders who saved 2 of 5 out-of-hospital cardiac arrest victims. In 1987, Cummins et al[22] reported a controlled study comparing the effectiveness of EMTs with AEDs and EMTs with manual defibrillators in treating 147 patients with VF in suburban Seattle, Washington. No statistically significant differences in rates of admission (54% AED; 50% manual) or survival to discharge (30% AED; 23% manual) were noted. In 1988, Weaver et al[13] reported on the use of AEDs primarily by non-EMT first responders (3.3-min response time) followed by paramedics (8.8-min response), compared with basic EMTs (3.4-min response) followed by paramedics (5.1-min response). A prototype AED was used and modified halfway through the study. The combined results of 504 patients with VF showed no difference in admission rates (59% AED; 53% EMT) but a higher rate of survival to discharge in the AED group (30% vs 19%). In 1987, Stults and Brown[23] reported on a study comparing AEDs used by EMTs with manual defibrillators used by EMTs. The results of 88 patients with VF showed no significant difference in rates of admission (29% AED; 32% manual) or survival to discharge (17% AED; 13% manual).

In Rochester, Minnesota (85 km$^2$, 76 000 inhabitants), White et al[24] established a system based on early defibrillation by police. In a total of 158 sudden death episodes, 84 were VF. Police intervened with a mean intervention time of 5.6 min compared to 6.3 min by paramedics ($P$=NS). Survival to discharge was 49% (41 of 84), with 18 of 31 (58%) in the police group and 23 of 53 (43%) in the paramedic group. A high discharge-to-home survival rate was obtained with early defibrillation

**Table 7.1** Percentage of survival rate in ventricular fibrillation patients. The total number of treated patients is given in parentheses.

| | % survival rate before early defibrillation program | % survival rate after early defibrillation program | Rate of survival increase |
|---|---|---|---|
| 1980 King County, Washington (8) | 7% | 26% (10/38) | 3.7 |
| 1984 Iowa (9) | 3% (1/31) | 19% (12/64) | 6.3 |
| 1986 Northestern Minnesota (10) | 2% (3/118) | 10% (8/81) | 5.0 |
| 1988 Southeast Minnesota (11) | 4% (1/27) | 17% (6/36) | 4.3 |
| 1984 Rural communities (12) | 3% (1/31) | 19% (12/64) | 6.3 |
| 1988 Seattle (13) | 19% (44/288) | 30% (84/276) | |
| 1989 Wisconsin (14) | 4% (32/983) | 11% (33/304) | 2.8 |
| 1998–2001 Indianapolis, Indiana (15) | 8% (16/204) | 10.6% (19/180) | 1.2 |
| 1996 Rochester, Minnesota (16) | — | 49% (41/84) | — |
| 1997 Munich (17) | — | 18.5% (45/243) | — |
| 1998 Pittsburgh (18) | 3% (1/29) | 26% (12/46) | 8.6 |
| 1998 Rochester, Minnesota (16) (19) | — | 40% (53/131) | — |
| 2002 Piacenza, Italy (20) | 21% (7/33) | 44% (15/34) | 2.1 |

by both police and paramedics with a short call-to-shock time. Even brief time decreases (e.g., 1 min) in call-to-shock time increase the likelihood of survival.

Bachman et al[25] failed to confirm the results from Iowa and Seattle in rural, northeastern Minnesota. They reported survival to discharge rates of 11% for paramedics, 5% for EMTs with manual defibrillators, and 2.5% for cardiac arrests handled by basic EMTs. Separate analysis for VF was not performed. They found no unwitnessed arrest survivors as earlier studies had, and the results caused them to question the use of AEDs in rural areas.

In contrast, Vukov[26] studied EMT defibrillation in rural southeastern Minnesota in 1988. In a report of 63 patients, EMTs with AEDs had significantly greater admission rates (30% vs 12%) and survival to discharge rates (17% vs 4%) than EMTs without AEDs.

A study from rural Tennessee in 1988 by Gentile et al[27] included 23 patients with VF treated by EMTs with AEDs. The average response time was 7.6 min. Survivors (9% of VF patients) were defibrillated within 4 min of collapse.

In 1982, Jaggarao et al[28] in the UK reported on 27 patients in cardiac arrest who were treated with AEDs and pacemakers in Brighton. Of this group, 15 patients had an initial rhythm of VF, one deteriorated to VF, and five (31%) survived to discharge. Of these, two had been treated with defibrillation and intubation. Three received both defibrillation and pacing during their resuscitation efforts. One patient with sinus tachycardia received a defibrillatory shock and degenerated to VF. He was able to return to a sinus rhythm after two further shocks. Two other patients were defibrillated inappropriately. Both were in a moving ambulance.

Gray et al reported using the Heart Aid on 65 patients with VF in Stockport in 1987.[29] Of the three (4.5%) patients admitted, none survived to discharge, despite an average response time of 4.5 min. He postulated that this was because fewer than a third had even rudimentary CPR.

*Present status of early defibrillation* The use of AEDs has become an important component of the EMS, and recent advances in AED technology have allowed expansion of AED use to nontraditional first responders and the lay public. The effectiveness of AEDs in this setting has been proven by several clinical trials.

Targeted responders (e.g., police) have effectively increased survival to hospital discharge by 14–58% by significantly decreasing the time to defibrillation.[30] A total of 193 patients presented with VF. Of these, 80 (41%) were discharged neurologically intact. Of the 159 VF patients whose arrest was bystander-witnessed, 73 (46%) were discharged. Survival from nonVF arrest was very low (5%). Assessment of VF survivors demonstrated a quality of life, adjusted for age, gender, and disease, similar to that of the general population.

Out-of-hospital cardiac arrest survival in suburban and rural Indiana did not improve after police were equipped with AEDs.[18] Even if intervals from 911 call-to-scene and 911 call-to-shock were shortened by 1.6 min and 4.8 min, respectively, for police response as compared with EMS response, survival to hospital discharge for VF out-of-hospital cardiac arrest was 15% (3/20) in cases in which police responded first, and 10% (16/160) in cases in which the EMS responded first ($P$=NS). Survival to hospital discharge for VF out-of-hospital cardiac arrest did not improve from the pre-study period mainly due to police poor response.

For patients with VF or ventricular tachycardia in Piacenza, Italy, the introduction of a two-tier system with first responders was associated with 44% survival to hospital discharge compared to 21% of medical staff alone.[20] The system serves a population of 173 114 residents. Equipment for the system comprised 39 AEDs: 12 placed in high-risk locations, 12 in lay-staffed ambulances, and 15 in police cars; 1285 lay volunteers trained in use of the AED, without training traditional CPR, responded to all cases of suspected SCD, in coordination with the EMS. During the first 22 months, 354 sudden cardiac death occurred (72±12 years, 73% witnessed). The Progetto Vita volunteers treated 143 SCD cases (40.4%), with an EMS call-to-arrival time of 4.8±1.2 min (vs 6.2±2.3 min for EMS, $P$= 0.05). Overall survival rate to hospital discharge was tripled from 3.3% (7 of 211) for EMS intervention to 10.5% (15 of 143) for lay volunteer intervention ($P$= 0.006). The survival rate for witnessed SCD was tripled by lay volunteers: 15.5% vs 4.3% in the EMS-treated group ($P$=0.002). A 'shockable' rhythm was present in 23.8% (34 of 143) of the Piacenza Progetto Vita (PPV) patients versus 15.6% (33 of 211) of the EMS patients ($P$=0.055). The survival rate from shockable dysrhythmia was higher for lay volunteers than EMS: 44.1% (15 of 34) versus 21.2% (7 of 33), $P$=0.046. The neurologically intact survival rate was higher in lay volunteer-treated than EMS-treated patients: 8.4% (12 of 143) versus 2.4% (5 of 211) ($P$=0.009).

Defibrillation by Casino security officers was associated with 35% survival to discharge[31] in Las Vegas, Nevada. The locations where the defibrillators were stored in the casinos were chosen to make possible a target interval of 3 min or less from collapse to the first defibrillation. The protocol called for a defibrillation first, followed by manual CPR. AEDs were used for 105 patients whose initial cardiac rhythm revealed VF. Fifty-six of the patients (53%) survived to discharge from the hospital. Among the 90 patients whose collapse was witnessed (86%), the clinically relevant time intervals were a mean of 3.5±2.9 min from collapse to attachment of the defibrillator, 4.4±2.9 min from collapse to the delivery of the first defibrillation shock, and 9.8±4.3 min from collapse to the arrival of the paramedics. The survival rate was 74% for those who received their first defibrillation no later than 3 min after a witnessed collapse and 49% for those who received their first defibrillation after more than 3 min.

The better innovation in the use of AEDs has been demonstrated in the Chicago Airport System HeartSave Project at O'Hare and Midway Airports,[32] where a new video system of self-instruction led to exciting results. AEDs were installed along passenger terminals at O'Hare, Midway, and Meigs Field airports, at a 60–90-s walk distance each from another. The use of defibrillators was promoted by public-service videos in waiting areas, pamphlets, and reports in the media. Over a 2-year period, 21 persons had sudden cardiac arrest, 18 of whom had VF. Eleven patients with VF were successfully resuscitated, including eight who regained consciousness before hospital admission. The rescuers, except for two, were good Samaritans acting voluntarily. Six of the 11 successfully resuscitated patients had no training or experience in the use of automated defibrillators, although three had medical degrees. Ten of the 18 patients with VF were alive and neurologically intact at 1 year.

In conclusion, pilot data in isolated populations suggest that volunteer non-medical responders can defibrillate safely and effectively, although no large-scale trials of such an approach have been conducted. No specific training seems to be necessary to use an AED safely and successfully. The role of CPR in a well-organized system of early defibrillation is of low priority importance.

### *3) Public access defibrillation: the future of early defibrillation*

In Europe, placement of AEDs in public places frequented by a large number of susceptible people will increase overall survival. However, placement of AEDs in all public places is still debatable, and further studies are necessary to estimate the potential impact of public access defibrillators. In the 5 years since the beginning of the project in Piacenza, Italy, there has been only one case of cardiac arrest where a publically placed AED was activated. In all other cases, police car AEDs were crucial for victims of cardiac arrest.

The Public Access Defibrillation (PAD) Trial[33] is a randomized, controlled trial designed to measure survival to hospital discharge following out-of-hospital cardiac arrest in community facilities with staff trained and equipped to provide PAD, compared to community facilities with staff trained to provide CPR without any capacity for defibrillation. The 2.5-year study has been conducted in 24 centers throughout North America. Some 19 000 volunteers in participating communities have been trained to recognize cardiac arrest, to access the 911 system, and to perform CPR. Half of the community units have AEDs placed in conspicuous locations, and the volunteers in those locations have been trained to use the devices. The AEDs have been placed in such community units as residential apartments, shopping centers, senior centers, gated communities, office buildings, and sports venues. Patients with treated out-of-hospital cardiac arrest in the two groups were similar in age (mean, 69.8 years), proportion of men (67%), rate of cardiac arrest in a public location (70%), and rate of witnessed cardiac arrest (72%). No inappropriate shocks were delivered. There were more survivors to hospital discharge in the units assigned to have volunteers trained in CPR plus the use of AEDs (30 survivors among 128 arrests) than there were in the units assigned to have volunteers trained only in CPR (15 among 107; $P=0.03$; relative risk, 2.0; 95% confidence interval, 1.07–3.77); there were only two survivors in residential complexes. This study and other smaller ones clearly indicate that implementation of community-based lay responder programs is feasible in many types of facilities, although these programs require resources, and many barriers to implementation of effective PAD programs still exist. In the PAD trial, volunteer attrition was high, 36% after 2 years.[34] Promoting citizen, fire department, and law enforcement response to sudden cardiac arrest remains an underappreciated yet critically important responsibility of public safety. We must help everyone in the community to understand that what they do in the first few minutes after witnessing someone's collapse has proven to be the most important determinant of victim future.

Barriers to implementation of public access defibrillation programs include a correct identification of 'high-risk' locations, lack of interest of the community, lack of motivated volunteer responders, training and retraining resource requirements, and lack of an existing communication and response infrastructure to coordinate the program.

The importance of timely defibrillation in persons in cardiac arrest has been established clearly by Stiell et al,[35] who reviewed data from the Ontario Prehospital Advance Life Support (OPALS) study for evidence to support this standard of care and the importance of early defibrillation. The OPALS study is a before-and-after clinical trial testing the benefit of adding rapid defibrillation and advanced life support to an existing basic life support system. The study includes 21 communities in Ontario served by 11 EMS programs.

Survivors of cardiac arrest were more likely to be young and to have a bystander-witnessed cardiac arrest and an initial rhythm of VF or tachycardia. A comparison of the response intervals with survival rates shows a steep decrease in the survival curve during the first 5 min, after which the slope gradually levels off. The curve shows that a 5-min response rate would have doubled the survival rate achieved with an 8-min target. The authors conclude that significant improvement in survival rates could be accomplished by decreasing the defibrillation response interval to less than 8 min. Patients in communities with EMS arrival times of less than 5 min have significantly better survival rates, thus strongly supporting the idea that early defibrillation is at the first step of the chain of survival.

### *4) Home defibrillation*

Since the majority of cardiac arrests occur at home, the obvious new frontier is home defibrillation. As defibrillators become smaller, less expensive and easier to use, the once futuristic idea of having defibrillators as common as fire extinguishers is no longer idle fancy (Figure 7.3 bottom).

The initial programs in home defibrillation actually began more than 15 years ago.[36] New AEDs have been approved for home use by untrained users. No prospective studies demonstrate that the use of AEDs in the home by untrained persons improves health outcomes. Further investigation is needed to determine the benefit of AEDs in the home.

Small, easy-to-use automatic defibrillators will soon rival the cost of home computers. This sort of defibrillation may be in the hands of everyone. Home defibrillators, along with an owner's manual and instructional video, are available to consumers only with a physician's prescription in the USA, and the US Food and Drug Administration is now deciding whether to permit the purchase of AEDs without a doctor's prescription. Individuals can buy a defibrillator online (www.CVS.com and www.americanaed.com), and they will soon become available for easy purchase at other Internet sources and even in local markets. It is conceivable that many individuals will buy their own defibrillator before these medical devices become routinely available at shopping malls, restaurants, churches, physicians' offices, health clubs, golf courses and other potentially high-risk locations. While academic issues are debated, the next frontier is clear: the personal use of defibrillators.

A recent study evaluated the use of AEDs in the home, businesses and other public settings by minimally trained first responders.[37] The study consisted of a telephone survey of businesses and public facilities (2683) and homes (145) owning at least one AED for at least 12 months. Thirteen percent (209/1581) of business and 5% (4/73) of home responders had used the AED for a suspected cardiac arrest. The rate of use for the AEDs was highest in residential buildings, public places, malls and recreational facilities, with an overall usage rate of 11.6% per year. In the four cases where the AED was used by a lay responder, all four patients survived to hospital admission and two were discharged from the hospital. There were no reports of injury or harm. In conclusion, this survey demonstrates that lay responders successfully used the AEDs in emergency situations with minimal training and with no reports of harm or injury to the operators, bystanders or patients.

## In-hospital defibrillation

Every year, an estimated 370 000–750 000 patients will have a cardiac arrest and undergo attempted resuscitation during their hospital stay. The rates of survival after in-hospital cardiac arrest average a low 15%, with similar rates even in closely monitored and staffed areas. In most instances, emergency care providers cannot get there fast enough to make a difference.

### *Results from in-hospital resuscitation efforts: variations in reported success*

For more than 30 years, researchers have published many studies on survival after in-hospital CPR. Until recently, no clear picture of success had emerged. Three major reviews of more than 50 published articles on survival after in-hospital CPR have demonstrated wide variations in survival. McGrath[38] calculated survival rates of 38% at 24 h (range 13–59%) and 15% at hospital discharge (range 3–27%). DeBard[39] reported survival rates of 39% at 24 h and 17% at discharge to home. Cummins and Graves[40] reviewed 44 studies and calculated survival rates to hospital discharge of 3–27% following an in-hospital cardiac arrest. Such wide variations in the rate of survival are explained largely by marked differences in inclusion criteria and outcome definitions.

Two large-scale projects provide the best evidence on success of in-hospital resuscitation. The Belgian Cardiopulmonary Cerebral Resuscitation Registry (BCCRR), working with the European Resuscitation Council, gathers information on survival from both in-hospital and out-of-hospital resuscitation.[41,42] In the British Hospital Resuscitation Study (BRESUS), investigators analyzed the results of 3765 attempted CPRs in 12 teaching and nonteaching hospitals throughout the UK.[43] Neither of these projects, however, is exclusively focused on in-hospital resuscitation. In BRESUS 25% of patients experienced onset of arrest during the prehospital phase. Investigators observed that 39% of patients survived the immediate arrest, 28% were alive 24 h later, 17% were discharged from the hospital, and 12.5% survived for 1 year. Both BRESUS and BCCRR helped pioneer standard methods of recording arrests for audit, clinical trials, and community studies.

The first-year experience with a hospital-wide first-responder AED programme implemented in a 683-bed university hospital.[44] Throughout the hospital, 14 'AED access spots' were identified which could be easily reached from all wards and diagnostic rooms within 30 s. AEDs were installed, and 120 medical officers, 750 nurses, and 50 administrative or technical staff underwent a 2-h training program. An AED was applied and activated by nurses/medical staff before the cardiac arrest team arrived in 27 of 33 cases (81.8%) of witnessed cardiac arrest. The median time from onset of the emergency call to the activation of the AED (record of ECG) was, on average, 2.1 min (range 1.0–4.5 min). In 18 of 27 cases in which the AED was installed promptly, the primary arrest rhythm was either ventricular tachycardia or VF, and the AED delivered a shock. For this subgroup, the rate of return of spontaneous circulation and the rate of discharge at home were 88.9 and 55.6%, respectively. This encourages us to extend the concept of first-responder AED defibrillation throughout the hospital.

## CONCLUSION

In conclusion, at the present time, programs for the use of AED exist only occasionally. The main reasons for this are the lack of open-mindedness, as well as logistic and legal problems. There have been no known lawsuits against lay rescuers providing CPR as good Samaritans, nor any against AED users. However, the perceived potential for a suit against a lay rescuer who used an AED has in some cases been a deterrent for companies or organizations considering establishing a public access defibrillation program. Today, airports, airlines, casinos, cruise ships, and other public venues that have modernized should have an AED in their first-aid kits. Although optimal placement of AEDs remains uncertain, public access defibrillation is showing great promise in reducing the death rate from sudden cardiac arrest. The lay public, both trained and untrained, is emerging as the next level of emergency care responders able to use a defibrillator. The future of public safety is defibrillation in the home. The strong collaboration between the EMS and a unique emergency call number is mandatory in Europe.

## REFERENCES


1. Cummins RO, Ornato JP, Thies WH, Pepe PE. Improving survival from sudden cardiac arrest: the 'chain of survival' concept. Circulation 1991; 83: 1832–47.
2. Cummins RO, Eisenberg MS, Hallstrom AP, Litwin PE. Survival of out-of-hospital cardiac arrest with early initiation of cardiopulmonary resuscitation. Am J Emerg Med 1985; 3: 114–19.
3. Eisenberg MS, Horwood BT, Cummins RO et al. Cardiac arrest and resuscitation: a tale of 29 cities. Ann Emerg Med 1990; 19: 179–86.
4. Becker LB, Ostrander MP, Barrett J, Kondos GT. Outcomes of CPR in a large metropolitan area – where are the survivors? Ann Emerg Med 1991; 20(4): 355–61.
5. Lombardi G, Gallagher J, Gennis P. Outcome of out-of-hospital cardiac arrest in New York City. The Pre-Hospital Arrest Survival Evaluation (PHASE) Study. JAMA 1994; 271(9): 678–83.
6. Watts DD. Defibrillation by basic emergency medical technicians: effect on survival. Ann Emerg Med 1995; 26: 635–9.
7. Mayfield T. EMS in the nation's most populous cities. J Emerg Med Serv 1998; 23: 51–69.
8. Eisenberg MJ, Copass MK, Hallstrom AP et al. Treatment of out of hospital cardiac arrest with rapid defibrillation by emergency medical technicians. N Engl J Med 1980; 302: 1379–83.

9. Stults KR, Brown DD, Schung VL, Bean JA. Prehospital defibrillation performance by emergency medical technicians in rural communities. N Engl J Med 1984; 310: 219–23.
10. Bachman JW, McDonald GS, O'Brien PC. A study of out-of-hospital cardiac arrests in northeastern Minnesota. JAMA 1986; 256: 477–83.
11. Vukov LF, White RD, Bachman JW et al. New perspective on rural EMT defibrillation. Ann Emerg Med 1988; 17: 318–21.
12. Ornato JP, McNeill SE, Craren EJ, Nelson NM. Limitation on effectiveness of rapid defibrillation by emergency medical technicians in a rural setting. Ann Emerg Med 1984; 12: 1096–9.
13. Weaver WD, Hill D, Fahrenbruch CE et al. Use of the automatic external defibrillator in the management of out-of-hospital cardiac arrest. N Engl J Med 1988; 319: 661–6.
14. Olson DL, LaRochelle J, Fark D et al. EMT-defibrillation. The Wisconsin experience. Ann Emerg Med 1989; 18: 806–11.
15. Groh WJ, Newman MM, Beal PE, Fineberg NS, Zipes DP. Limited response to cardiac arrest by police equipped with automated external defibrillators: lack of survival benefit in suburban and rural Indiana – the Police as Responder Automated Defibrillation Evaluation (PARADE). Acad Emerg Med 2001; 8: 324–30.
16. White RD, Asplin BR, Bugliosi TF, Hankins DG. High discharge survival rate after out-of-hospital ventricular fibrillation with rapid defibrillation by police and paramedics. Ann Emerg Med 1996; 28: 480–5.
17. Ladwig KH, Schoefinius A, Danner R et al. Effects of early defibrillation by ambulance personnel on short- and long-term outcome of cardiac arrest survival: the Munich experiment. Chest 1997; 112: 1584–91.
18. Mosesso VN, Davis EA, Auble TE et al. Use of automatic external defibrillators by police officers for treatment of out-of-hospital cardiac arrest. Ann Emerg Med 1998; 32(2): 200–7.
19. White RD, Hankins DG, Bugliosi TF. Seven years' experience with early defibrillation by police and paramedics in an emergency medical services system. Resuscitation 1998; 39: 145–51.
20. Capucci A, Aschieri D, Piepoli MF et al. Tripling survival from sudden cardiac arrest via early defibrillation without traditional education in cardiopulmonary resuscitation. Circulation 2002; 106(9): 1065–70.
21. Chadda KD, Kammerer R. Early experiences with the portable automatic external defibrillator in the home and public places. Am J Cardiol 1987; 60(8): 732–3.
22. Cummins RO, Eisenberg MS, Litwin PE et al. Automatic external defibrillators used by emergency medical technicians. A controlled clinical trial. JAMA 1987; 257(12): 1605–10.
23. Stults KR, Brown DD, Cooley F, Kerber RE. Self-adhesive monitor/defibrillation pads improve prehospital defibrillation success. Ann Emerg Med 1987; 16(8): 872–7.
24. White RD, Asplin BR, Bugliosi TF, Hankins DG. High discharge survival rate after out-of-hospital ventricular fibrillation with rapid defibrillation by police and paramedics. Ann Emerg Med 1996; 28(5): 480–5.
25. Bachman JW, McDonald GS, O'Brien PC. Study of out-of-hospital cardiac arrests in northeastern Minnesota. JAMA 1986; 256(4): 477–83.
26. Vukov LF, White RD, Bachman JW, O'Brien PC. New perspectives on rural EMT defibrillation. Ann Emerg Med 1988; 4: 318–21.
27. Gentile D, Auerbach P, Gaffron J, Foon G, Phillips J Jr. Prehospital defibrillation by emergency medical technicians. Results of a pilot study in Tennessee. J Tenn Med Assoc 1988; 81(3): 144–8.
28. Jaggarao NS, Heber M, Grainger R et al. Use of an automated external defibrillator-pacemaker by ambulance staff. Lancet 1982; 2(8289): 73–5.
29. Gray AJ, Redmond AD, Martin MA. Use of the automatic external defibrillator-pacemaker by ambulance personnel: the Stockport experience. BMJ (Clin Res Ed) 1987; 294(6580): 1133–5.
30. White RD, Bunch TJ, Hankins DG. Evolution of a community-wide early defibrillation programme experience over 13 years using police/fire personnel and paramedics as responders. Resuscitation 2005; 65(3): 279–83.

31. Valenzuela TD, Roe DJ, Nichol G et al. Outcomes of rapid defibrillation by security officers after cardiac arrest in casinos. N Engl J Med 2000; 343: 1206–9.
32. Caffrey SL, Willoughby PJ, Pepe PE, Becker LB. Public use of automated external defibrillators. N Engl J Med 2002; 347(16): 1242–7.
33. Hallstrom AP, Ornato JP, Weisfeldt M et al. Public-access defibrillation and survival after out-of-hospital cardiac arrest. N Engl J Med 2004; 351(7): 637–46.
34. Richardson LD, Gunnels MD, Groh WJ et al. PAD Trial Investigators. Implementation of community-based public access defibrillation in the PAD trial. Acad Emerg Med 2005; 12(8): 688–97.
35. Stiell IG, Wells GA, Field B et al. Ontario Prehospital Advanced Life Support Study Group. Advanced cardiac life support in out-of-hospital cardiac arrest. N Engl J Med 2004; 351(7): 647–56.
36. Eisenberg MS, Cummins RO. Automatic external defibrillation: bringing it home. Am J Emerg Med 1985; 3(6): 568–9.
37. Jorgenson DB, Skarr T, Russell JK, Snyder DE, Uhrbrock K. AED use in businesses, public facilities and homes by minimally trained first responders. Resuscitation 2003; 59(2): 225–33.
38. McGrath RB. In-house cardiopulmonary resuscitation: after a quarter of a century. Ann Emerg Med 1987; 16: 1365–8.
39. DeBard M. Cardiopulmonary resuscitation: analysis of six years experience and review of the literature. Ann Emerg Med 1981; 1: 408–16.
40. Cummins R, Graves J. Clinical results of standard CPR: pre-hospital and in-hospital. In: Kaye W, Bircher NG, eds. Cardiopulmonary Resuscitation. New York: Churchill Livingstone, 1989: 87–102.
41. Forms for registration of CPR efforts and outcome, respectively, for out-of-hospital and in-hospital cardiac arrest. Prepared by the Working Group on Research Coordination of the European Resuscitation Council, in collaboration with the Cerebral Resuscitation Study Group of the Belgian Society for Emergency and Disaster Medicine and the Working Group on CPR of the European Academy of Anaesthesiology. Resuscitation 1992; 24: 155–66.
42. Cerebral Resuscitation Study Group. The Belgian Cardiopulmonary Cerebral Resuscitation Registry: form protocol. Resuscitation 1989; 17(Suppl): S5–10.
43. Tunstall-Pedoe H, Bailey L, Chamberlain DA et al. Survey of 3765 cardiopulmonary resuscitations in British hospitals (the BRESUS study): methods and overall results. BMJ 1992; 304: 1347–51.
44. Hanefeld C, Lichte C, Mentges-Schroter I, Sirtl C, Mugge A. Hospital-wide first-responder automated external defibrillator programme: 1 year experience. Resuscitation 2005; 66(2): 167–70.

# 8

# New guidelines on first aid in cardiac arrest

Alessandro Capucci and Daniela Aschieri

Cardiac arrest is a medical emergency that, if left untreated, invariably leads to death within a few minutes. A cardiac arrest is the cessation of normal circulation of the blood due to failure of the heart to contract effectively during systole. Cerebral hypoxia causes victims to lose consciousness immediately and stop breathing. The primary first-aid treatment for cardiac arrest is *cardiopulmonary resuscitation (CPR)*, which is defined as emergency first aid for an unconscious person on whom breathing and pulse cannot be detected. First aid is a series of simple, life-saving medical techniques that a layman can be trained to perform. However, even when performed correctly, CPR can injure the person it is performed on. This is a normal occurrence, and should always be taken into account. When an automatic external defibrillator (AED) is present, it can be considered a first-aid device to be used by bystanders and certainly the most promising intervention.

Since CPR was first proposed in the early 1960s, resuscitation science has continued to advance, and clinical guidelines have been updated regularly to reflect these developments and advise healthcare providers on best practice. They provide for clearance of the airway, intermittent positive pressure ventilation, and chest compression as essential interventions. This chapter contains the guidelines for adult CPR by lay rescuers and guidelines for the use of an AED updated to the new International Guidelines for Resuscitation 2005.[1,2]

## MAIN CHANGES IN NEW 2005 GUIDELINES ON FIRST AID

The most significant change to CPR guidelines is related to the ratio of chest compressions to rescue breaths – from 15 compressions for every two rescue breaths in the 2000 International Guidelines to 30 compressions for every two rescue breaths in the 2005 International Guidelines. The 30:2 ratio is the same for CPR that a single lay rescuer provides to adults, children and infants (excluding newborns).

Another guidelines change emphasizing the importance of CPR is the sequence of rhythm analysis and CPR in using an AED. Previously, when AED pads were applied to the chest, the device analyzed the heart rhythm, delivered a shock if necessary, and analyzed the heart rhythm again to determine whether the shock successfully stopped the abnormal rhythm. The cycle of analysis, shock and re-analysis could be repeated three times before CPR was recommended, resulting in delays of 37 s or more. Now, after one shock, the new guidelines recommend that rescuers provide about 2 min of CPR, beginning with chest compression, before activating the AED to reanalyze the heart rhythm and attempt another shock. Studies have shown that the first AED shock stops the abnormal cardiac arrest rhythm more than 85% of the time and that a brief period of chest compressions between shocks can deliver oxygen to the heart, increasing the likelihood of successful defibrillation.

The guidelines also recommend that healthcare providers minimize interruptions to chest compressions by doing heart rhythm checks, inserting airway devices, and administering of drugs without delaying CPR.

The new recommendations continue to encourage greater implementation of AED programs in public locations like airports, casinos, sports facilities and businesses. The 2005 guidelines reflect the results of the Public Access Defibrillation Trial, which reinforced the importance of planned and practiced response to cardiac emergencies by lay rescuers.

The new guidelines recommend that 911 dispatchers should be trained to provide CPR instructions by phone and help callers correctly identify cardiac arrest victims. Dispatchers may talk rescuers through compressions-only CPR for most adult victims of cardiac arrest; however, instructions to do compressions and rescue breaths will also be given for infants and children or adult victims of asphyxia caused by near-drowning or other noncardiac causes. Dispatchers also should be trained to recognize the symptoms of heart attack and other acute coronary syndromes, and advise such patients to chew an aspirin while awaiting response by the EMS.

These guidelines do not define the 'only way that resuscitation should be achieved', as underlined by some authors: they represent a widely accepted view of how resuscitation can be undertaken both safely and effectively. In particular, the publication of these new and revised treatment recommendations does not imply that current clinical care is either unsafe or ineffective. The European Resuscitation Council Executive Committee considers these new recommendations to be the most effective and easily learned interventions that can be supported by current knowledge, research and experience.

## THE IMPORTANCE OF CPR

The brain is the main organ to suffer from oxygen depletion, and it may sustain irreversible damage after about 6 min. Following cardiac arrest, effective CPR enables enough oxygen to reach the brain to delay brain death, and allows the heart to remain responsive to defibrillation attempts. CPR is hardly ever effective if started more than 15 min after collapse, because permanent brain damage has probably already occurred. A notable exception is cardiac arrest occurring with exposure to very cold temperature.

CPR is commonly taught to ordinary people, who may be the only ones present in the crucial few minutes before emergency personnel are available. CPR is never guaranteed to save life. Almost 35 years have elapsed since the combined techniques of mechanical ventilation and external precordial compression were introduced in clinical practice. External defibrillation ushered in the modern era of CPR. Even if CPR intervention may generate sufficient alveolar ventilation for few minutes, the outcome after 'sudden death' is very disappointing if defibrillation is not performed within 5 min after collapse. Less than 3% of sudden cardiac death victims (SCD) are likely to undergo resuscitation with return to an optimal level of functioning within this time.

## CHEST COMPRESSION THEORY

Closed chest cardiac massage was first described in 1878 by Boehm and successfully applied in a few cases of cardiac arrest over the next 10 years or so. CPR was developed by Peter Safar in the 1950s, and he wrote the book *The ABC of Resuscitation* in 1957. After that, 1960 could be considered the year in which modern CPR was born. Early marketing efforts oversold the effectiveness of CPR in rescuing heart attack and other victims.

The original term 'cardiac massage' and its successor 'external cardiac compression' reflect the initial theory as to how chest compressions achieve an artificial circulation by squeezing the heart. This 'heart-pump theory' was criticized in the mid-1970s; firstly, because echocardiography demonstrated that the cardiac valves become incompetent during resuscitation and, secondly, because coughing alone was shown to produce a life-sustaining circulation. The alternative 'thoracic pump' theory proposes that chest compression, by increasing intrathoracic pressure, propels blood out of the thorax, because veins at the thoracic inlet collapse while the arteries remain patent.

The recommended rate of 100 compressions/min reflects a compromise between scientific evidence in favor of faster compression, and the ability of the rescuers to maintain the higher speeds. It is important, however, to recognize that, even when performed optimally, chest compressions do not achieve more than 30% of the normal cerebral perfusion. Interruptions of chest compressions must be minimized. On stopping chest compression, the coronary flow decreases substantially; on resuming chest compression, several compressions are necessary before the coronary flow recovers to its previous level.[3] Recent evidence indicates that unnecessary interruptions of chest compressions occur frequently, both in- and out-of-hospital.[4–6] Resuscitation instructors must emphasize the importance of minimizing interruptions of chest compressions.

## THE ALGORITHM OF CPR FOR ADULTS

The adult basic resuscitation algorithm reported in Figure 8.1 has been updated to reflect changes in the European Resuscitation Council and American Heart Association guidelines. Rescuers begin CPR if the victim is unconscious or unresponsive, and not breathing normally (ignoring occasional gasps). A single compression–ventilation (CV) ratio of 30:2 is used for the single rescuer of an adult or child (excluding neonates) out of hospital, and for all adult CPR. This single ratio has been designed to simplify teaching, promote skill retention, increase the number of compressions given and decrease interruption of compressions. Once a defibrillator is attached, if a shockable rhythm is confirmed, a single shock is delivered. The most significant change in the protocol is that, irrespective of the resultant rhythm, chest compressions and ventilations (2 min with a CV ratio of 30:2) are resumed immediately after the first shock to minimize the 'no-flow' time. Once the airway is secured with a tracheal tube, laryngeal mask airway or Combitube, the lungs are ventilated at a rate of 10 per min without pausing during chest compressions. Adult CPR is appropriate for children over 8 years old.

### Approaching the patient

The first step in the CPR procedure is to ensure that there is no danger to any person involved before the patient is approached. The rescuer comes in front of the patient, gently shakes his shoulders and asks loudly: 'Can you hear me?', 'Are you all right?' If there is a response, the rescuer leaves the patient in the original position, provided there is no further danger; and tries to find out what is wrong with him; and

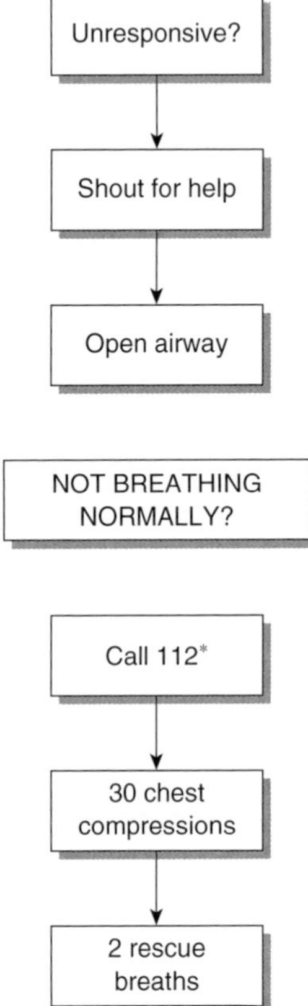


*Or other national emergency number

**Figure 8.1** Adult basic life-support algorithm.

summons help if needed. If there is no response, a single rescuer will generally need to call for help before starting CPR.

### Calling for help

The call for help in first aid is only a step of the emergency action procedure, typically made after assessing the scene. Current practice is to telephone for help and to supply information on the state of victims as requested by the emergency operator.

With any telephone anywhere in the world, one can call an emergency number for assistance. These numbers include:

- 118 in Italy
- 000 in Australia
- 111 in New Zealand
- 112 can be used in addition to any local emergency number within the European Union and on GSM cellular phone networks worldwide.
- 119 in parts of Asia
- 911 in North America

- 991 in Malaysia
- 999 in the UK, a number of Commonwealth countries and Hong Kong.

Various international emergency telephone numbers are reported at www.sccfd.org/travel.html. If the local emergency number is unknown, one should try the four most popular variations 999, 911, 112 and 119. When connected to the emergency service, the proper procedure is for callers to:

1. Identify themselves.
2. Give the phone number from which they are calling, if they are asked for it. This will allow callback in case the communication is interrupted. A phone number can also physically locate the caller. In many cases, the operator will know the number from which the call originates, as it is often passed on automatically by the telephone network.
3. Give the *exact* location of the event, including the name of the city, the name of the building, or the number of the street, and its direction.
4. Describe the situation, illness or accident, and in the last case, specifics of the incident and the number of casualties.
5. When there are only a few casualties, describe general state (alert or unalert, breathing or not) and the affliction (physical trauma, disease, or other).
6. List the first-aid actions already performed.
7. Answer the questions, and listen to the information given; *never hang up first*.

## The ABC

The three elements of basic life support after assessment of the situation are commonly remembered as 'ABC': *Airway/Breathing/Circulation*.

### *A for airway*

Quick inspection of the mouth may reveal a blocked airway. If possible, the patient should be placed on his back on a firm surface. The next step is to get a further view of the mouth and throat and to make as much space for breathing as possible:

- In a neck injury, lifting the chin or jaw may be enough to stabilize the airway;
- In other cases, tilting the head back will lift the tongue away from the back of the mouth, opening the airway.

### *B for breathing*

Look, listen and feel for no more than 10 s to determine whether the victim is breathing normally. After opening the victim's airway, check breathing effort. Place your cheek in front of the victim's mouth (about 3–5 cm away), while looking at the chest and gently put your hand on the chest of the patient; this should allow you to detect any of the following signs:

1. feeling the airflow on the cheek
2. hearing the airflow
3. feeling the chest rise and fall
4. seeing the chest rise and fall.

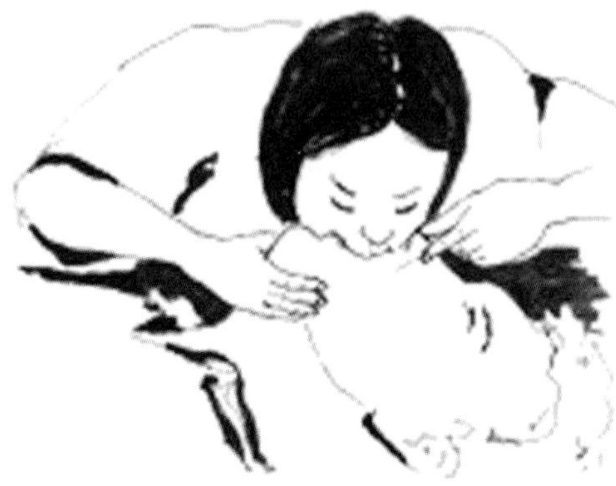

**Figure 8.2** Mouth-to-mouth rescue breathing. The head of the patient is tilted backward. The rescuer closes the patient's nose with one hand, while lifting the chin with her other hand to keep the mouth open.

If there is no breathing, or the patient does not breath normally (gasping), start artificial respiration.

Rescue breathing is the act of mechanically forcing air into a patient's respiratory system; it is indicated *only* in respiratory arrest, and *not* in a weakly breathing patient (Figure 8.2). Ideally, you should *never* blow into an unknown person's body for fear of projections of bodily fluids (blood, vomit, etc.); thus, if you have a CPR mask, or even a cotton handkerchief, use it to protect yourself.

A CPR mask allows insufflation but prevents the rescuer from being exposed to the patient's exhaled air or body fluids (such as vomit), as well as direct connection to an oxygen bottle. Start by giving two insufflations. These can help a nearly breathing patient recover spontaneous respiration. Table 8.1 reports the main recommendation for a breathing rescuer.

***Artificial respiration: HOW TO DO IT ....***

- Tilt back the head of the patient to extend his airways.
- Open the jaw of the patient by pulling on his chin. In some cases (like some cases of epilepsy), the muscles of patients are so contracted that it is impossible to open the mouth. Contrary to urban legend, patients will not 'swallow' their tongues. In this situation, it may not be possible to blow into the mouth. Instead, seal the lips together and breath into the nose while keeping the head tilted back.
- Close the nose of the patient with your free hand.
- Take a deep breath, put your mouth on the mouth of the patient in an airtight manner, and blow into the mouth of the patient. These breaths should be gentle and last no longer than 2 s to prevent air from entering the stomach.

Therefore, the current recommendation is for rescuers to give each rescue breath about 1 s, with enough volume to make the victim's chest rise (500 ml tidal volume is considered enough), but to avoid rapid or forceful breaths. This recommendation applies to all forms of ventilation during CPR, including mouth-to-mouth and bag-valve-mask with and without supplementary oxygen. Mouth-to-nose ventilation is an effective alternative to mouth-to-mouth ventilation. When you have given two

| **Table 8.1** Rescue breathing: Recommendations from the 2005 guidelines |
|---|
| 1. During CPR, blood flow to the lungs is substantially reduced, so an adequate ventilation : perfusion ratio can be maintained with lower tidal volumes and respiratory rates than normal. |
| 2. Hyperventilation (too many breaths or too large a volume) is not only unnecessary, but also harmful, because it increases intrathoracic pressure, thus decreasing venous return to the heart and diminishing cardiac output. Survival is consequently reduced. |
| 3. When the airway is unprotected, a tidal volume of 1 l produces significantly more gastric distention than a tidal volume of 500 ml. |
| 4. Low minute-ventilation (lower than normal tidal volume and respiratory rate) can maintain effective oxygenation and ventilation during CPR. During adult CPR, tidal volumes of approximately 500–600 ml (6–7 ml/kg) should be adequate. |
| 5. Interruptions in chest compression (as to give rescue breaths) have a detrimental effect on survival. Giving rescue breaths over a shorter time will help to reduce the duration of essential interruptions. |

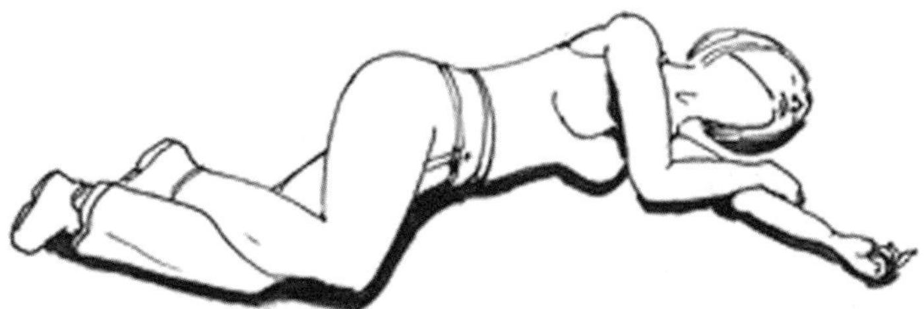

**Figure 8.3** The recovery position. Note that various forms of this position are taught, and the position shown here differs from that described in the text, but the principles are similar. The mouth is downward so that vomit or blood can drain from the patient; the chin is well up to keep the epiglottis open. Arms and legs are locked to stabilize the position of the patient.

insufflations, check for signs of circulation, while keeping an eye on the patient's respiration. There are two possibilities:

- The patient might have recovered spontaneous respiration thanks to your insufflations.
- The patient might be in a state of cardiorespiratory arrest.

If the patient has recovered spontaneous respiration, put him in the recovery position (Figure 8.3).

If the patient is in a state of cardiorespiratory arrest, you will have to perform cardiac massage.

The recovery position is a first-aid technique recommended to protect the airway of an unconscious person, so that the person can breathe.

***The recovery position: HOW TO DO IT…***
The following steps describe how to put someone in the recovery position. Note that even if the exact steps are not remembered, it is still generally much better to turn unconscious victims onto their side than to leave them on their back.

- Put yourself in a position where you will be pulling the person toward you. Your own body can serve as a brake if the person's weight is more than you can control as you turn him.
- Place the arm closest to you with right angles at both the shoulder and the elbow, in a 'hand-up' position.
- Raise the knee of the far leg. The foot of the far leg should end up flat on the ground, approximately next to the knee of the near leg.
- Bring the hand of the far arm against the person's near cheek (palm outward) and support it with your hand.
- Turn the person onto their side by gently pulling the raised knee/thigh of the far leg, while continuing to hold the person's hand against their cheek with your other hand, thereby supporting the head.
- When you have the person on their side, tilt the head back to ensure an open airway, adjusting the position of the arms as necessary to support the head in this position. Check the person's breathing.
- For maximum stability, position the upper leg so that there are right angle bends at both the hip and the knee.

*C for circulation*

The 'gold standard' sign of cardiac arrest is an absent carotid (or other large artery) pulse. Other methods of checking for circulation vary, and are taught in line with the accepted teaching in a particular organization or country. A layperson is advised to check for 'signs of circulation' such as color in the skin or movements such as breathing, coughing or twitching, for no more than 10 s.

Therefore, lay people should be taught to begin CPR if the victim is unconscious (unresponsive) and not breathing normally. It should be emphasized during training that agonal gasps occur. Checking the carotid pulse is now considered an inaccurate method of confirming the presence or absence of circulation.[7] In an emergency situation, there is not usually time to check for pulse, especially for lay rescuers. Some experts no longer advise laypersons to assess the carotid pulse because it wastes time and studies have shown that it leads to an incorrect conclusion in up to 50% of cases. Instead, they recommend looking for other visible signs of circulation. Health professionals are still advised to perform a carotid pulse check, taking no more than 10 s, whilst also checking the other signs of a circulation. However, there is no evidence that checking for movement, breathing or coughing is diagnostically superior. This may be because the airway is not open[8] or because the victim is making occasional (agonal) gasps. Bystanders often misinterpret agonal gasps as normal breathing. This can result in the bystander withholding CPR from a cardiac arrest victim.[9] Agonal gasps are present in up to 40% of cardiac arrest victims.[10] They are an indication to start CPR immediately and should not be confused with normal breathing. Healthcare professionals as well as lay rescuers also have difficulty in determining

| **Table 8.2** Rescue chest compression: recommendation from the 2005 guidelines |
|---|
| 1. Each time compressions are resumed, the rescuer should place his hands without delay 'in the center of the chest'. |
| 2. Compress the chest at a rate of about 100 compressions per min. Pay attention to achieving the full compression depth of 4–5 cm (for an adult). |
| 3. Allow the chest to recoil completely after each compression. |
| 4. Take approximately the same amount of time for compression and relaxation. |
| 5. Minimize interruptions to chest compression. |
| 6. Do not rely on a palpable carotid or femoral pulse as a gauge of effective arterial flow. |

the presence or absence of adequate or normal breathing in unresponsive victims[11,12] commonly in the first few minutes after cardiac arrest.

In any event, if there is no breathing, coughing or movement after the rescue breaths but there is circulation, continue rescue breathing. Check for signs of circulation regularly, as the patient might fall into cardiac arrest at any time. If there is no circulation, begin chest compressions.

Table 8.2 reports the main recommendation for chest compression.

***Chest compression: HOW TO DO IT …***
After having performed two insufflations,

- Place the victim on their back on a firm surface.
- Kneel next to the victim's chest.
- Remove, open or cut away the patient's clothes. CPR must be performed close to the patient's chest.
- Place your hands directly above the sternum, one on top of the other, two fingers' width above the point where the lower ribs meet (Figure 8.4). To avoid injuring the ribs, only the heel of your hand should touch the chest 'in the center of the chest, between the nipples'.[13] It has been shown that for healthcare professionals the same hand position can be found more quickly if rescuers are taught to 'place the heel of your hand in the center of the chest with the other hand on top', provided the teaching includes a demonstration of placing the hands in the middle of the lower half of the sternum.[13] It is reasonable to extend this to lay people.
- It is especially important to avoid making compressions at the exact point where the ribs meet in order to avoid breaking the xiphoid process, as this could cause tremendous damage to the lungs or other internal organs.
- Shift your weight forward on your knees until your shoulders are directly over your hands.
- Keeping your elbows locked straight, repeatedly bear down and then come up, bear down and come up. You must depress the chest of an average adult about 4–5 cm with each compression.[14]
- It is important to release completely after each chest compression.[15]
- Compress the chest about 100 times every minute.[16–18]
- Try to compress and release for equal periods of time.

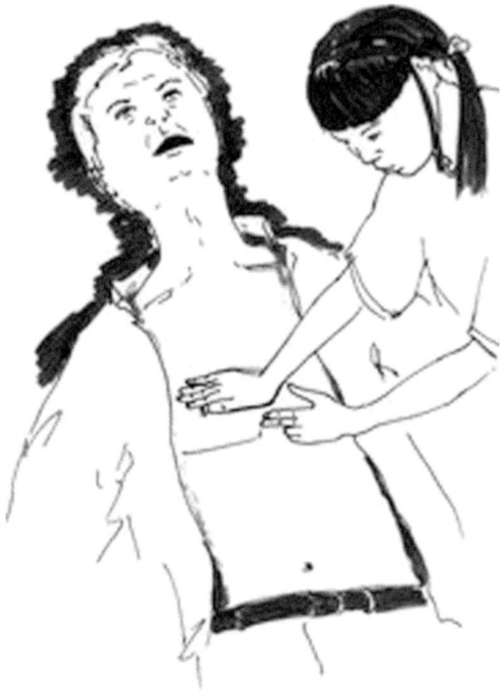

**Figure 8.4** Positioning the hand before giving CPR. The hand must be placed two fingers away from where the ribs meet (the xiphoid process).

- After 30 compressions, open the airway again by head tilt and chin lift.
- Give the victim two rescue breaths.
- Return to the victim's chest and put your hands in the correct position again.
- Repeat this cycle of 30 and two, and stop to recheck the victim only if he starts breathing normally; otherwise, do not interrupt resuscitation.
- Do not rely on a palpable carotid or femoral pulse as a gauge of effective arterial flow.[19]
- If there is more than one rescuer present, another should take over CPR every 1–2 min to prevent fatigue. Ensure the minimum of delay during the changeover of rescuers.

With conventional external precordial compression, we try to restore systemic blood flow. However, CPR, even when well performed, generates cardiac outputs that represent less than 30% of normal values. In animal models, systolic arterial pressure peaks at 60–80 mmHg, diastolic pressure remains low, and mean arterial pressure in the carotid artery seldom exceeds 40 mmHg. The benefit of chest compression is especially important if the first shock is delivered more than 5 min after collapse, since it generates a small but critical amount of blood flow to the brain and myocardium and increases the likelihood that defibrillation will be successful.

Accordingly, several alternatives to conventional precordial compression have been proposed with the aim of increasing cardiac output and both coronary and cerebral blood flows. These include interposed abdominal compression, active decompression, circumferential chest compression, intermittent ascending aortic balloon occlusion, extracorporeal circulation, and, most recently, phased chest and abdominal compression–decompression.

## MAIN LIMITATION IN PERFORMING CPR

In the era of public access defibrillation, the main (probably the only one) object of our efforts should be to reduce time to defibrillation. This may be done only by increasing the number of AEDs in the community. Too much money and effort are still spent in training people to perform CPR. In the last 20 years, the only communities that have demonstrated an increase in neurologically damage-free survival have been those with well-established, early defibrillation programs. In recent guidelines, too much importance has been given to CPR training, which is too limited and should be considered a marginal support of early defibrillation. The examples of Seattle, Rochester, Piacenza, Chicago and Las Vegas have clearly demonstrated the necessity of access to an AED within 5 min, as the guidelines recommend. How many communities provide this? How many EMS administrators spend time and economic resources to establish such a community project? Very few, if any, communities have developed a strategic program in this way. The common strategy is to equip ambulances with defibrillators, without considering that the only rescuers who can quickly reach victims of SCD are police or public AED. This two-tier system (police cars and public access defibrillators) should be considered strictly a part of the EMS, not, as now, as a still marginal branch of a failing, ambulance-based emergency system.

The major limitation of this approach to new guidelines is to create a great dependence on CPR by lay responders while their potential role in defibrillation is still exceptional.

It is well recognized that skill acquisition and retention are aided by simplification of the CPR sequence of actions.[20] In particular, it is too easy to use AED alone rather than to perform correctly CPR. CPR should be considered for ambulance rescuers, not for all lay rescuers.

In fact, if not performed correctly, ventilation may be detrimental. During adult CPR, tidal volumes of approximately 500–600 ml (6–7 ml/kg) should be adequate.[21–24] As recommended in the new guidelines, if ventilation is performed with too many breaths or too large a volume, it may be harmful because it increases intrathoracic pressure, thus decreasing venous return to the heart and diminishing cardiac output. Survival is consequently reduced. A tidal volume of 1 l produces significantly more gastric distention than a tidal volume of 500 ml.

Moreover, lay rescuers as well as healthcare professionals are often reluctant to perform mouth-to-mouth ventilation on unknown victims of cardiac arrest.[25–27] This is a major limitation when CPR is performed by laypersons, especially if we think of the cost of continuous training in the community. For these reasons, and to emphasize the priority of chest compressions, new guidelines recommend that CPR in adults should start with chest compression rather than initial ventilation, thus modifying protocol with no ventilation at all. Is this enough to maintain brain perfusion? No human studies exist on this, as much of the information about the physiology of chest compression and the effects of varying the compression rate, compression-to-ventilation ratio, and duty cycle (ratio of time chest is compressed to total time from one compression to the next) is derived from animal models.

### Risk to the rescuers

The safety of both rescuer and victim is paramount during a resuscitation attempt.[28] There have been a few incidents of rescuers suffering adverse effects from undertaking CPR, with only isolated reports of infections such as tuberculosis[29] and severe acute respiratory distress syndrome (SARS).[30] Transmission of HIV during CPR has never been reported. There have been no human studies to address the effectiveness of barrier devices during CPR; however, laboratory studies have shown that certain filters, or barrier devices with one-way valves, prevent oral bacterial transmission from the victim to the rescuer during mouth-to-mouth ventilation.[31] Rescuers should take appropriate safety precautions where feasible, especially if the victim is known to have a serious infection, such as tuberculosis or SARS.[32] During an outbreak of a highly infectious condition, such as SARS, full protective precautions for the rescuer are essential.

### Compression-only CPR

Healthcare professionals as well as lay rescuers admit to being reluctant to perform mouth-to-mouth ventilation on unknown victims of cardiac arrest.[33] Animal studies have shown that chest compression-only CPR may be as effective as combined ventilation and compression in the first few minutes after nonasphyxial arrest.[34] In adults, the outcome of chest compression without ventilation is significantly better than the outcome of giving no CPR. If the airway is open, occasional gasps and passive chest recoil may provide some air exchange. A few minute-ventilations may be all that is necessary to maintain a normal ventilation-perfusion ratio during CPR.

Therefore, lay people should be encouraged to perform compression-only CPR if they are unable or unwilling to provide rescue breaths, although combined chest compression and ventilation is a better method of CPR.

#### *D for defibrillation*

The first AED was described in 1979.[35] This defibrillator incorporated a digital computer-based rhythm analysis system for automatic diagnosis of shockable rhythm. The defibrillation electrodes serves dual functions of transducing the ECG signals and delivery of the transthoracic electric shock. When ventricular fibrillation (VF) or ventricular tachycardia is recognized and confirmed by the software, the device is sequenced to charge its capacitor and deliver one countershock. The rhythm is re-evaluated, and the capacitor is recharged for the next countershock. Initial experience has been encouraging. The AED may be the most important advance in improving outcomes of out-of-hospital CPR. It is in the setting of out-of-hospital cardiac arrest, and specifically sudden death, that the need is most urgent. Unless defibrillation is accomplished within the critical time interval (3–5 min in the absence of bystander CPR or within 8 min if CPR is initiated promptly and correctly), the

**Table 8.3** The safe use of AEDs: recommendations from the 2005 guidelines

1. Take off any oxygen mask and nasal cannulae and place them at least 1 m away from the patient's chest.
2. Leave the ventilation bag connected to the tracheal tube or other airway adjunct. Alternatively, disconnect any bag-valve device from the tracheal tube (or other airway adjunct such as the laryngeal mask airway, Combitube or laryngeal tube), and move it at least 1 m from the patient's chest during defibrillation.
3. If the patient is connected to a ventilator, as in the operating room or critical care unit, leave the ventilator tubing (breathing circuit) connected to the tracheal tube unless chest compressions prevent the ventilator from delivering adequate tidal volumes. In this case, the ventilator is usually replaced with a ventilation bag, which can itself be left connected or detached and removed to a distance of at least 1 m. If the ventilator tubing is disconnected, ensure it is kept at least 1 m from the patient or, better still, switch the ventilator off; modern ventilators generate massive oxygen flows when disconnected. During normal use, when connected to a tracheal tube, oxygen from a ventilator in the critical care unit will be vented from the main ventilator housing well away from the defibrillation zone. Patients in the critical care unit may be dependent on positive end expiratory pressure (PEEP) to maintain adequate oxygenation; during cardioversion, when the spontaneous circulation potentially enables blood to remain well oxygenated, it is particularly appropriate to leave the critically ill patient connected to the ventilator during shock delivery.
4. Minimize the risk of sparks during defibrillation. Theoretically, self-adhesive defibrillation pads are less likely to cause sparks than manual paddles.

likelihood of successful resuscitation is remote. First responders may now include defibrillation with AEDs as part of their CPR.

Public access to AEDs has been strongly recommended by all international guidelines. The general public must be trained in the use of the AEDs if we are to reduce the number of sudden deaths. Public emergency services typically cannot respond within the critical time window of 5 min.

## New guidelines

The main change proposed by the European Society of Cardiology (ESC) guidelines on the AED algorithm is to delivery a single shock and without reassessing the rhythm or feeling for a pulse, resume CPR (30 compressions : two ventilations) for 2 min before delivering another shock (if indicated). This recommendation is based mainly on two observations: 1) in the three-shock protocol (as recommended in the 2000 guidelines) if the patient is refractory to the first shock, the time before CPR is about 80 s; 2) the first-shock efficacy have been reported to be no more than 10%.[36–39] The ESC Commission considers that these observations indicate the need of a period of CPR rather than a further shock. Even if animal studies show that these delays greatly compromise the success of the resuscitation attempt,[40–42] there are no published human or animal studies comparing a single-shock protocol with a three-stacked-shock protocol for treatment of VF cardiac arrest. Thus, immediately after giving a single shock, and without reassessing the rhythm or feeling for a pulse, the new 2005 guidelines suggest resumption of CPR (30 compressions : two ventilations) for 2 min before delivering another shock (if indicated).

Table 8.3 reports the main recommendations for the safe use of AED.

> ***Defibrillation: HOW TO DO IT ...***
> As soon as the defibrillator arrives,
>
> - Switch on the defibrillator and attach the electrode pads. If more than one rescuer is present, CPR should be continued while this is carried out.
> - Follow the spoken/visual directions.
> - Ensure that nobody touches the victim while the AED is analyzing the rhythm (Figure 8.5).
>
> If a shock is indicated,
>
> - Ensure that nobody touches the victim.
> - Push shock button as directed (AEDs will deliver the shock automatically).
> - After the shock, continue to perform CPR 30:2 for 2 min.
> - Continue as directed by the voice/visual prompts.
>
> If no shock is indicated,
>
> - Immediately resume CPR, using a ratio of 30 compressions to two rescue breaths.
> - Continue as directed by the voice/visual prompts.
>
> Continue to follow the AED prompts until:
>
> - Qualified help arrives and takes over.
> - The victim starts to breathe normally.
> - You become exhausted.

Standard AEDs are suitable for use in children older than 8 years. For children of 1–8 years, use pediatric pads or a pediatric mode if available; if these are not available, use the AED as it is. Use of AEDs is not recommended for children under 1 year.

The sequence of action during defibrillation with the AED is guided by the voice/visual prompt. Any change from the 2000 guidelines involves changes in the voice and visual message of AEDs that guide the user of an AED through the procedure. AED vocal and visual messages are nowadays focused on the electrical defibrillation process and do not integrate with ventilation and chest compression indication, as requested by the 2005 guidelines.

According to the new guidelines, the vocal message should be reprogrammed as follows:

1. a single shock only, when a shockable rhythm is detected
2. no rhythm check, or check for breathing or a pulse, after the shock
3. a voice prompt for immediate resumption of CPR after the shock (giving chest compressions in the presence of a spontaneous circulation is not harmful)
4. two minutes for CPR before a prompt to assess the rhythm, breathing or a pulse is given.

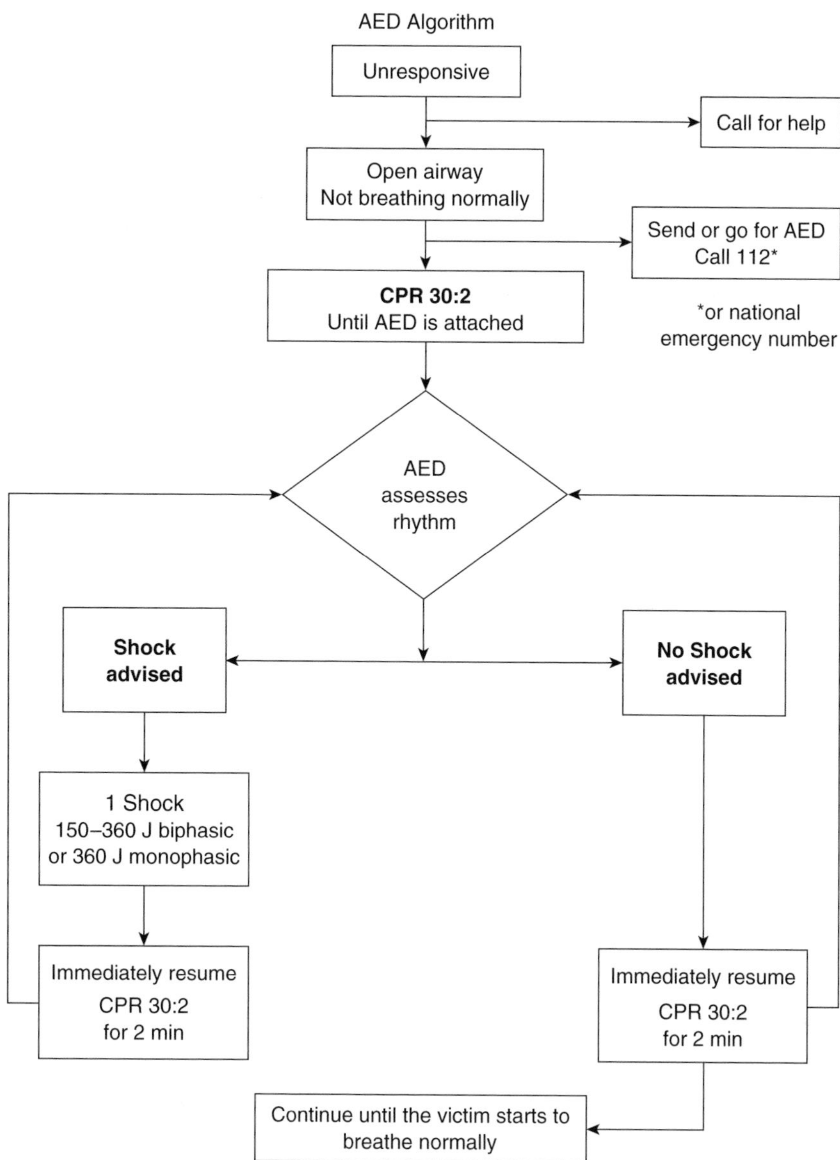


**Figure 8.5** Algorithm for the use of AED.

## CPR before defibrillation

Even if some evidence[43–45] supports a period of CPR before defibrillation as beneficial for survival, new guidelines recommend an immediate shock, as soon as the AED is available. In fact, CPR in these studies was performed by paramedics, who protected the airway by intubation and delivered 100% oxygen (such high-quality ventilation cannot be expected from lay rescuers giving mouth-to-mouth ventilation). The benefit seems to be present when AED arrives greater than 5 min after collapse. One study[46] did not confirm this benefit. In clinical practice, the delay from collapse to arrival is rarely known, and if bystander CPR is already in progress when the AED arrives, it is not logical to continue it.

### Fully automatic AEDs

Having detected a shockable rhythm, a fully automatic AED will deliver a shock without further input from the rescuer. One manikin study showed that untrained nursing students committed fewer safety errors with a fully automatic AED than a semi-automatic AED. There are no human data to determine whether these findings can be applied to clinical use.

## REFERENCES

1. 2005 American Heart Association Guidelines for Cardiopulmonary Resuscitation and Emergency Cardiovascular Care. Circulation 2005; 112(24) Suppl.
2. Handley AJ, Koster R, Monsieurs K et al. European Resuscitation Council Guidelines for Resuscitation 2005. Section 2. Adult basic life support and use of automated external defibrillators. Resuscitation 2005; 67 Suppl 1: S7–23.
3. Kern KB, Hilwig RW, Berg RA, Ewy GA. Efficacy of chest compression-only BLS CPR in the presence of an occluded airway. Resuscitation 1998; 39: 179–88.
4. Wik L, Kramer-Johansen J, Myklebust H et al. Quality of cardiopulmonary resuscitation during out-of-hospital cardiac arrest. JAMA 2005; 293: 299–304.
5. Abella BS, Alvarado JP, Myklebust H et al. Quality of cardiopulmonary resuscitation during in-hospital cardiac arrest. JAMA 2005; 293: 305–10.
6. Abella BS, Sandbo N, Vassilatos P et al. Chest compression rates during cardiopulmonary resuscitation are suboptimal: a prospective study during in-hospital cardiac arrest. Circulation 2005; 111: 428–34.
7. Bahr J, Klingler H, Panzer W, Rode H, Kettler D. Skills of lay people in checking the carotid pulse. Resuscitation 1997; 35: 23–2.
8. Domeier RM, Evans RW, Swor RA, Rivera-Rivera EJ, Frederiksen SM. Prospective validation of out-of-hospital spinal clearance criteria: a preliminary report. Acad Emerg Med 1997; 4: 643–6.
9. Hauff SR, Rea TD, Culley LL et al. Factors impeding dispatcher-assisted telephone cardiopulmonary resuscitation. Ann Emerg Med 2003; 42: 731–7.
10. Clark JJ, Larsen MP, Culley LL, Graves JR, Eisenberg MS. Incidence of agonal respirations in sudden cardiac arrest. Ann Emerg Med 1992; 21: 1464–7.
11. Ruppert M, Reith MW, Widmann JH et al. Checking for breathing: evaluation of the diagnostic capability of emergency medical services personnel, physicians, medical students, and medical laypersons. Ann Emerg Med 1999; 34: 720–9.
12. Perkins GD, Stephenson B, Hulme J, Monsieurs KG. Birmingham assessment of breathing study (BABS). Resuscitation 2005; 64: 109–13.
13. Handley AJ. Teaching hand placement for chest compression – a simpler technique. Resuscitation 2002; 53: 29–36.
14. Wik L, Kramer-Johansen J, Myklebust H et al. Quality of cardiopulmonary resuscitation during out-of-hospital cardiac arrest. JAMA 2005; 293: 299–304.
15. Yannopoulos D, McKnite S, Aufderheide TP et al. Effects of incomplete chest wall decompression during cardiopulmonary resuscitation on coronary and cerebral perfusion pressures in a porcine model of cardiac arrest. Resuscitation 2005; 64: 363–72.
16. Yu T, Weil MH, Tang W et al. Adverse outcomes of interrupted precordial compression during automated defibrillation. Circulation 2002; 106: 368–72.

17. Swenson RD, Weaver WD, Niskanen RA, Martin J, Dahlberg S. Hemodynamics in humans during conventional and experimental methods of cardiopulmonary resuscitation. Circulation 1988; 78: 630–9.
18. Kern KB, Sanders AB, Raife J et al. A study of chest compression rates during cardiopulmonary resuscitation in humans: the importance of rate-directed chest compressions. Arch Intern Med 1992; 152: 145–9.
19. Ochoa FJ, Ramalle-Gomara E, Carpintero JM, Garcia A, Saralequi I. Competence of health professionals to check the carotid pulse. Resuscitation 1998; 37: 173–5.
20. Handley JA, Handley AJ. Four-step CPR – improving skill retention. Resuscitation 1998; 36: 3–8.
21. Idris A, Gabrielli A, Caruso L. Smaller tidal volume is safe and effective for bag-valve-ventilation, but not for mouth-to-mouth ventilation: an animal model for basic life support. Circulation 1999; 100 Suppl I: I–644.
22. Idris A, Wenzel V, Banner MJ, Melker RJ. Smaller tidal volumes minimize gastric inflation during CPR with an unprotected airway. Circulation 1995; 92 Suppl: I–759.
23. Dorph E, Wik L, Steen PA. Arterial blood gases with 700 ml tidal volumes during out-of-hospital CPR. Resuscitation 2004; 61: 23–7.
24. Winkler M, Mauritz W, Hackl W et al. Effects of half the tidal volume during cardiopulmonary resuscitation on acid–base balance and haemodynamics in pigs. Eur J Emerg Med 1998; 5: 201–6.
25. Brenner BE, Van DC, Cheng D, Lazar EJ. Determinants of reluctance to perform CPR among residents and applicants: the impact of experience on helping behavior. Resuscitation 1997; 35: 203–11.
26. Ornato JP, Hallagan LF, McMahan SB, Peeples EH, Rostanfinski AG. Attitudes of BCLS instructors about mouth-to-mouth resuscitation during the AIDS epidemic. Ann Emerg Med 1990; 19: 151–6.
27. Hew P, Brenner B, Kaufman J. Reluctance of paramedics and emergency medical technicians to perform mouth-to-mouth resuscitation. J Emerg Med 1997; 15: 279–84.
28. Mejicano GC, Maki DG. Infections acquired during cardiopulmonary resuscitation: estimating the risk and defining strategies for prevention. Ann Intern Med 1998; 129: 813–28.
29. Sepkowitz KA. Occupationally acquired infections in health care workers. I. Ann Intern Med 1996; 125: 826–34.
30. Christian MD, Loutfy M, McDonald LC et al. on behalf of the SARS Investigation Team. Possible SARS coronavirus transmission during cardiopulmonary resuscitation. Emerg Infect Dis 2004; 10(2): 287–93.
31. Weiss SH. Risks and issues for the health care worker in the human immunodeficiency virus era. Med Clin North Am 1997; 81: 555–75.
32. Risk of infection during CPR training and rescue: supplemental guidelines. The Emergency Cardiac Care Committee of the American Heart Association. JAMA 1989; 262: 2714–5.
33. Jelinek GA, Gennat H, Celenza T, O'Brien D, Jacobs I, Lynch D. Community attitudes towards performing cardiopulmonary resuscitation in Western Australia. Resuscitation 2001; 51(3): 239–46.
34. Hallstrom A, Cobb L, Johnson E, Copass M. Cardiopulmonary resuscitation by chest compression alone or with mouth-to-mouth ventilation. N Engl J Med 2000; 342: 1546–53.
35. Diack AW, Welbom WS, Rullman RG et al. An automatic cardiac resuscitator for emergency treatment of cardiac arrest. Med Instrum 1979; 13: 78–82.
36. Bain AC, Swerdlow CD, Love CJ et al. Multicenter study of principles-based waveforms for external defibrillation. Ann Emerg Med 2001; 37: 5–12.
37. Poole JE, White RD, Kanz KG et al. Low-energy impedance-compensating biphasic waveforms terminate ventricular fibrillation at high rates in victims of out-of-hospital cardiac arrest. LIFE investigators. J Cardiovasc Electrophysiol 1997; 8: 1373–85.
38. Schneider T, Martens PR, Paschen H et al. Multicenter, randomized, controlled trial of 150-J biphasic shocks compared with 200- to 360-J monophasic shocks in the resuscitation of out-of-hospital cardiac arrest victims. Optimized Response to Cardiac Arrest (ORCA) Investigators. Circulation 2000; 102: 1780–7.

39. Rea TD, Shah S, Kudenchuk PJ, Copass MK, Cobb LA. Automated external defibrillators: to what extent does the algorithm delay CPR? Ann Emerg Med 2005; 46: 132–41.
40. Berg RA, Sanders AB, Kern KB et al. Adverse hemodynamic effects of interrupting chest compressions for rescue breathing during cardiopulmonary resuscitation for ventricular fibrillation cardiac arrest. Circulation 2001; 104: 2465–70.
41. Kern KB, Hilwig RW, Berg RA, Sanders AB, Ewy GA. Importance of continuous chest compressions during cardiopulmonary resuscitation: improved outcome during a simulated single lay-rescuer scenario. Circulation 2002; 105: 645–9.
42. Yu T, Weil MH, Tang W et al. Adverse outcomes of interrupted precordial compression during automated defibrillation. Circulation 2002; 106: 368–72.
43. Cobb LA, Fahrenbruch CE, Walsh TR et al. Influence of cardiopulmonary resuscitation prior to defibrillation in patients with out-of-hospital ventricular fibrillation. JAMA 1999; 281: 1182–8.
44. Wik L, Hansen TB, Fylling F et al. Delaying defibrillation to give basic cardiopulmonary resuscitation to patients with out-of-hospital ventricular fibrillation: a randomized trial. JAMA 2003; 289: 1389–95.
45. Eftestol T, Wik L, Sunde K, Steen PA. Effects of cardiopulmonary resuscitation on predictors of ventricular fibrillation defibrillation success during out-of-hospital cardiac arrest. Circulation 2004; 110: 10–15.
46. Jacobs IG, Finn JC, Oxer HF, Jelinek GA. CPR before defibrillation in out-of-hospital cardiac arrest: a randomized trial. Emerg Med Australas 2005; 17: 39–45.

# 9

# Post-resuscitation care

Erga L Cerchiari and Federico Semeraro

Post-resuscitation care includes all the diagnostic, therapeutic and prognostic interventions indicated in the treatment of patients resuscitated from cardiac arrest. Interventions range from early monitoring to prevent recurrence and searching for reversible causes of arrest to the long-term intensive care aimed at restoration of optimal cerebral and overall outcome – cardiopulmonary cerebral resuscitation.[1]

From a clinical perspective, after resuscitation from cardiac arrest, patients either recover consciousness or remain unconscious as a function of the duration of cardiac arrest and cardiopulmonary resuscitation (CPR), taking into account pre-arrest conditions such as age and comorbidities.[2]

It has long been believed that outcome is mostly, if not exclusively, determined by events occurring during cardiac arrest and CPR. For this reason, in the last 20 years, the focus of research and investment has been on identifying means to grant the timely interventions required to restore spontaneous circulation, the so-called chain of survival.[3]

Shortening the duration of cardiac arrest and CPR definitely improves the chances of successful resuscitation with optimal outcome; that is, the patient immediately recovers consciousness.

However, the widespread application of resuscitation techniques to reverse clinical death has led to increasingly frequent observations of a pathologic condition occurring in the patient who remains unconscious following resuscitation after prolonged cardiac arrest.

This condition, the post-resuscitation syndrome (PRS), exhibits the combination of whole-body ischemia and reperfusion as a unique pathogenetic determinant, and is characterized by a 'sepsis-like' condition with increased acute-phase response proteins, high levels of circulating cytokines, adhesion molecules, leukocyte dysregulation and plasma endotoxin, associated with multiple-organ dysfunction, primarily cerebral and myocardial.[4]

To reduce the occurrence of unfavorable outcome of resuscitation from cardiac arrest, efforts have been devoted to identify predictors of survival measurable during cardiac arrest and CPR efforts, and to develop scoring systems to be utilized by rescuers to interrupt CPR efforts. However, all these scores are difficult to apply when responding to patients in cardiac arrest and do not take into account the quality of post-resuscitation care.

The relevance of the quality of post-resuscitation in-hospital treatment and its impact on overall outcome after resuscitation from cardiac arrest has been confirmed by two clinical studies showing that factors associated with better outcome encompassed pre-arrest patient conditions (age under median 71 years and better overall performance category pre-arrest) and pre-hospital care (shorter call receipt by EMS to CPR interval and no use of epinephrine) but also in-hospital care. The absence of seizure activity, temperature, glucose levels and acidemia during the early post-resuscitation phase positively correlated with outcome.[5–6]

Furthermore, definitive evidence of the importance of post-resuscitation care in outcome has been provided by the landmark studies showing that moderate therapeutic hypothermia, induced after restoration of spontaneous circulation, significantly improves long-term survival and neurologic outcome.[7]

The rational for applying therapeutic interventions early after reperfusion from cardiac arrest is to interfere with the injurious mechanisms triggered by the cardiac arrest that continue to evolve during reperfusion and impair recovery from the initial ischemic–hypoxic damage induced by cardiac arrest.

Coronary reperfusion strategies, performed early after resuscitation, improve myocardial recovery and function and reduce the recurrence of cardiac arrest during the post-resuscitation phase.

Therefore, to improve the dismal survival rate of cardiac arrest patients, besides optimizing the timeliness and quality of emergency response, effort should be devoted to improve the quality of post-resuscitation care early after reperfusion and maintain it until reliable prognostication of the quality of long-term outcome can be achieved and meaningful decisions on further therapeutic strategies can be formulated.

This chapter will focus on post-resuscitation events, review the dimensions of the problem, review the etiopathogenetic mechanisms as the basis for treatment, and analyze the clinical pictures and therapeutic strategies.

## THE DIMENSION OF THE PROBLEM

The incidence of out-of-hospital cardiac arrest is estimated at 49.5–66 per 100 000 subjects per year.[2] The majority of these patients die outside the hospital, but return of spontaneous circulation leading to admission to hospital can be achieved in 17–33%, according to the efficiency of the emergency response system.[8] This means that the number of patients requiring post-resuscitation care after out-of-hospital cardiac arrest may range from 125 to 200 per million inhabitants per year.

The incidence of in-hospital cardiac arrest has been measured in 1.4/100 admissions/year;[9] in these, restoration of spontaneous circulation is 40–44%,[10] so that the number of patients requiring post-resuscitation care after in-hospital cardiac arrest is comparable to that of out-of-hospital cardiac arrest.

Of the patients resuscitated from cardiac arrest, a small fraction (variable as a function of timeliness and effectiveness of response) is of optimal recovery, awake and breathing spontaneously: identifying and treating the cause of arrest appear to be the main, if not the sole, therapeutic challenge for this group of subjects.

Since most survivors of cardiac arrest (80%) are comatose post-resuscitation, they are admitted to the intensive care unit (ICU) and represent the PRS population, which can be estimated at 15–20% of the total cardiac arrest victims.[11]

Among the PRS patients, mortality has been reported to be very high, reaching 80% by 6 months post-resuscitation.[12,13] Approximately one-third of the deaths are due to cardiac causes (early deaths usually <24 h), one-third to extracerebral organ malfunction, and one-third to neurologic causes (late deaths).

## ETHIOPATHOGENESIS

The damage occurring during cardiac arrest and CPR is multifaceted, encompassing several contributing pathogenetic factors:

- ischemia–anoxia during the no-flow condition occurring during cardiac arrest
- hypoperfusion–hypoxia during the low-flow condition, generated by external cardiac compressions.

The damage induced is a function of the duration of cardiac arrest and CPR.

Restoration of spontaneous circulation stops the progression of the ischemic insults and grants survival. However, during reperfusion, a variety of pathologic mechanisms triggered by cardiac arrest develop that may add to the initial insult and impair recovery.

Two major pathogenetic pathways have been identified:

1. direct insult to the brain, which is particularly sensitive to ischemia; and to the heart, which may suffer post-resuscitation myocardial stunning that, in turn, may lead to a secondary insult from post-reperfusion impairment of cardiac output and hypoperfusion
2. post-reperfusion activation of the systemic inflammatory response syndrome, with hypoperfusion and/or altered perfusion as a major pathologic determinant.[4]

Starting with reperfusion, major changes occur in hemodynamics, perfusion and organ function; three major phases have been identified.[1,11,14]

1. *an immediate phase* (first 30 min) of hemodynamic instability, characterized by cerebral and overall hyperperfusion (resulting from dishomogeneous cerebral distribution of flow), vasoparalysis and acid washout
2. *an early phase* (from 30 min to 4–6 h post-reperfusion) of cerebral and overall hypoperfusion associated with a dishomogeneous cerebral flow distribution maintaining areas of anaerobic metabolism (During this phase, significant clotting disturbances and activation inflammatory mediators are described.)
3. *a delayed phase* (after 6 h to 2–3 days post-reperfusion) of normalization of cardiovascular parameters accompanied by the development of organ dysfunction. (This phase shares many features with the multiple-organ dysfunction syndrome described in severe sepsis.)

## FACTORS AFFECTING OUTCOME AFTER INITIAL RESUSCITATION

The quality of survival after cardiac arrest is affected by pre-arrest, arrest and post-resuscitation variables, which are different for out-of-hospital and in-hospital cardiac arrest.

The analysis of factors associated with survival of out-of-hospital cardiac arrest showed a correlation with pre-arrest variables, such as increasing age, history of diabetes, or heart failure, as well as with variables related to the events of arrest and quality of response, including initial rhythm, witnessed arrest, bystander CPR, time to first defibrillation, and the duration of cardiac arrest.[15]

The analysis of factors associated with survival of in-hospital cardiac arrest showed a correlation with pre-arrest variables including pre-arrest sepsis, metastatic cancer, dementia, African-American race, serum creatinine level, cancer, coronary artery disease and location of arrest.[16]

After pre-hospital resuscitation, the patient's status at admission to the hospital is an important determinant of outcome, underlying the relevance of the quality of post-resuscitation care during the pre-hospital post-resuscitation phase: this includes level of consciousness,[15] presence of cardiogenic shock[17] and presence of sinus rhythm.

The relevance of the quality of in-hospital treatment and its impact on overall outcome after resuscitation from cardiac arrest has been confirmed by the finding that among resuscitated patients, the mortality rate differs significantly between hospitals.[5] Factors associated with better outcome include the condition of patients pre-arrest (age under median 71 years and better overall performance category pre-arrest), prehospital care (shorter call receipt by EMS to CPR interval and no use of epinephrine), and in-hospital care (no seizure activity, temperature under 37.8°C (median), S-glucose under 10.6 mmol/l 24 h after admission (median), and persisting acidosis (median base excess greater than 3.5 mmol/L) 12 hours after admission.

In another recent study, Skrifvars et al[6] identified as associated with outcome, age, delay before the return of spontaneous circulation, mean blood glucose and serum potassium, and the use of beta-blocking agents during post-resuscitation care.

## CLINICAL FEATURES

From a clinical perspective, after resuscitation from cardiac arrest, patients either recover consciousness or remain unconscious as a function of the duration of cardiac arrest and CPR, and of pre-arrest conditions such as age and comorbidities.

Usually, during the first hour post-reperfusion, two clinical pictures may be delineated clearly:

1. *The awake patient*: following brief durations of arrest, the patient gradually regains consciousness and spontaneous breathing. The patient may still be confused, but responds to pain and to simple verbal command.
2. *The unconscious patient*: following more prolonged durations of cardiac arrest, the patient remains comatose, i.e., does not response to painful stimulation, and requires assisted ventilation.

In all patients resuscitated from cardiac arrest, the priority is to identify and treat the cause of arrest and support, as needed, cardiovascular function, which may be impaired as a result of arrest or of the underlying cause of arrest, in order to prevent recurrence.

Beyond the cardiac-oriented interventions, treatment strategies differ, and awake and comatose patients require increasing complexity of care.

## TREATMENT STRATEGIES

Treatment strategies vary according to the clinical picture of the single patient and to the different post-resuscitation phases (Figure 9.1).

- Immediate post-resuscitation care aims to stabilize the patient and support vital functions in order to prevent recurrence of cardiac arrest, and to ensure safe transportation to the hospital for out-of-hospital cardiac arrest, and to the final level of care for in-hospital cardiac arrest. Regardless of patient status, the provider of care should support adequate airways and breathing, administer

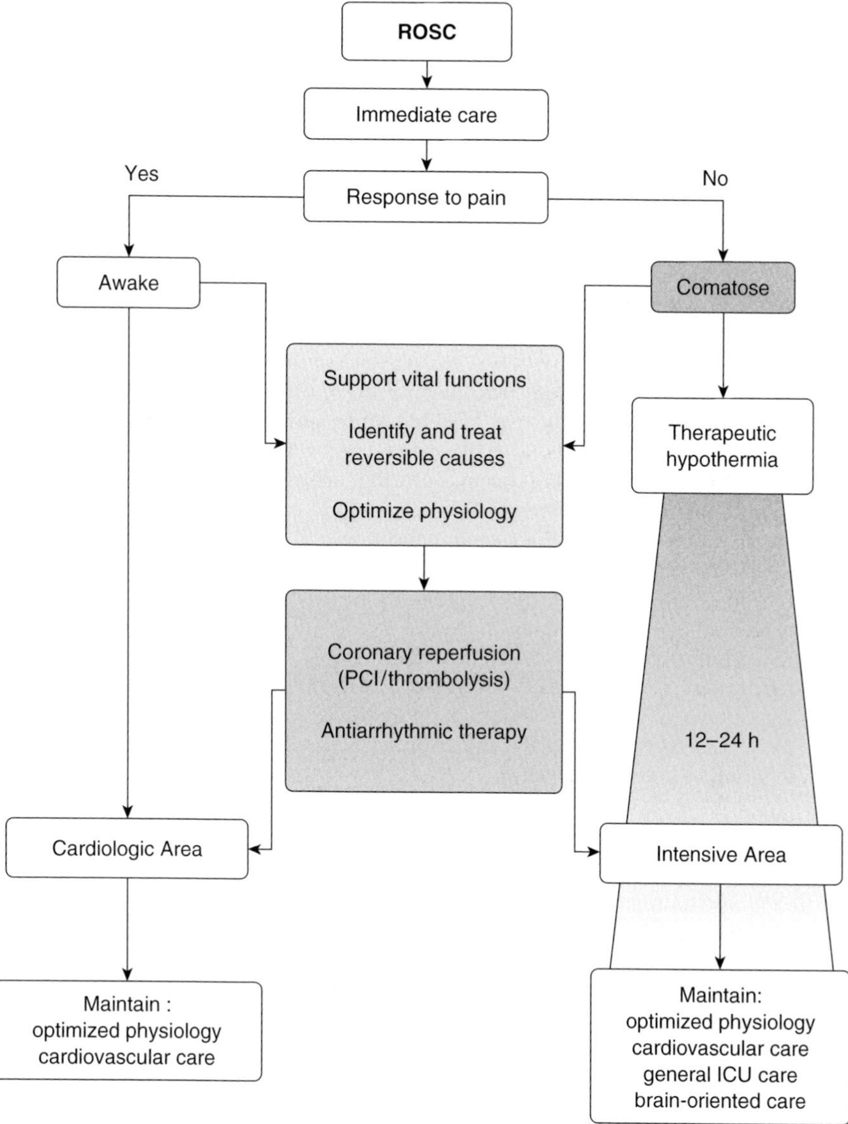


**Figure 9.1** The post-resuscitation therapeutic options are related to the patient condition and to the phases of care ranging from immediate (on-scene) to early time-dependent interventions (in gray) to long term (until 24–72 h post-ROSC).

supplemental oxygen, monitor the patient's vital signs, and establish or verify existing intravenous access.

- Early post-resuscitation care includes the support of vital functions as needed and the identification and treatment of reversible causes of arrest. In this phase, 30 min after establishing restoration of spontaneous circulation (ROSC), response to painful stimulation allows one to distinguish between patients who will shortly awake from those who will remain comatose. The support of vital functions for the comatose patient includes support of airways and breathing (artificial ventilation may be necessary) and optimization of physiology, including oxygen saturation, acidosis and cardiovascular function. During this phase, time-dependent treatments should be initiated, including beta blockade in arrests of presumed cardiac origin, coronary reperfusion strategies (thrombolysis or percutaneous coronary intervention (PCI) based on duration of symptoms, ECG, contraindications and available facilities), and hypothermia in comatose patients (with sedation and ventilation). As soon as feasible, optimization of physiology should be started.

- Following the time-dependent interventions, post-resuscitation care differs in awake and comatose patients, and patients require admission to differentiated levels of care as follows:

  - *Awake patient*: a patient responding to painful stimuli, after coronary revascularization if indicated, beta blockade and exclusion of other reversible causes of arrest/effects of CPR, needs to be admitted to an intermediate cardiologic level of care for monitoring against recurrence of arrest, and maintenance of cardiovascular care and optimized physiology until stabilization of the cardiovascular condition.
  - *Comatose patient*: a patient not responding to painful stimuli, after starting hypothermia, coronary revascularization if indicated, beta blockade and exclusion of other reversible causes of arrest/effects of CPR, must be admitted to an intensive level of care to monitor against recurrence of arrest; maintain cardiovascular care and optimized physiology; and initiate/continue hypothermia requiring sedation, ventilation and neuromuscular blockade, prompt seizures treatment, and optimal ICU care until a reliable prognostic evaluation becomes possible.

## THERAPEUTIC INTERVENTIONS

The single therapeutic options are grouped below in four categories (optimize physiology, cardiac-oriented interventions, general ICU care and brain-oriented interventions), and the available evidence to support each option is based on the recent review process performed in the ILCOR consensus on science, and the analysis utilizes the same criteria.[18–21] In relation to the post-resuscitation phase, the time to initiation and the estimated duration of the single theraputic options are arbitrarily summarized for mnemonic purposes in Table 9.1.

### Optimize physiology

The treatment of the patient resuscitated from cardiac arrest should focus on maintaining within normal ranges all the physiologic variables, the alteration of which may facilitate the recurrence of cardiac arrest or unfavorably affect neurologic recovery.

#### *Cardiovascular function*

Hemodynamic instability is common after restoration of spontaneous circulation and manifests as hypotension, low cardiac index and arrhythmia. There are very few randomized trials evaluating the role of blood pressure on the outcome after cardiac arrest. One randomized study, although showing no difference between

**Table 9.1** Therapeutic interventions post-resuscitation. Bold face indicates high level of evidence – strongly recommended intervention. The times indicate the phase in which the intervention should be started/the duration for which the intervention should be maintained

| Post-resuscitation care reminders | Awake | Comatose |
|---|---|---|
| **Immediate care** | | |
| Support airway | | |
| Support breathing/administer oxygen | Regardless of patient status | |
| Monitor patient (ECG, *Pa*, $Sa_{O_2}$) | | |
| Establish and verify intravenous access | | |
| **Identify/treat cause of arrest and CPR complications** | **Early/intermediate** | |
| **Cardiac-oriented interventions** | | |
| **Beta-blockers** | **Early** | |
| **Coronary reperfusion therapy (thrombolysis/PCI)** | **Early** | |
| Amiodarone if beta-blockers is not tolerated | Early | |
| **ICD therapy** | **Late** | |
| **Optimize physiology** | | |
| avoid temperatures over 37°C | Intermediate/prolonged | |
| Normalize serum $Mg^{2+}$ and $K^{+}$ level | Early/prolonged | |
| Treat hyperglycemia and avoid hypoglycemia | Intermediate | **Intermediate/prolonged** |
| Correct severe acidosis | Early | Early/Prolonged |
| $Fi_{O_2}$ to achieve $Pa_{O_2}$ > 100 mmHg for 24 h ($Sa_{O_2}$ of 99–100%) | Intermediate | Intermediate/prolonged |
| Maintain blood pressure | **Early/prolonged** | |
| **General ICU** | | |
| Ventilation, sedation and neuromuscular blockade | | Early/prolonged until hypothermic |
| Ventilation to normocarbia – avoid hypocarbia | | Early/prolonged |
| **Brain-oriented interventions** | | |
| Treat seizure following cardiac arrest | | Promptly |
| **Hypothermia 32–34°C in ROSC after VF** | | **Early/prolonged** |
| Hypothermia 32–34°C in ROSC after nonshockable rhythms | | Early/prolonged |

patients randomized to > 100 vs < 100 mmHg at 5 min post-ROSC, revealed that arterial blood pressure during the first 2 h post-resuscitation was independently and positively associated with good functional neurologic recovery, whereas hypotensive episodes correlated with poor cerebral outcome.[22] The post-resuscitation myocardial dysfunction (or global myocardial stunning) is usually transient, being more prolonged and severe as a function of the duration of cardiac arrest and resuscitation efforts,[23,24] as well as the contribution of the amount of epinephrine utilized during CPR,[17,25] and correlates to the levels of circulating proinflammatory cytokines.[17] Myocardial dysfunction, the echocardiographic monitoring of which may be useful in this phase, improves at 24–48 h post-resuscitation with return to normal values, although with persisting superimposed vasodilation: persistently low cardiac index at 24 h post-resuscitation was associated with early death by multiple-organ failure, but not with neurologic outcome.[17] Successful treatment of myocardial dysfunction is essential to reduce the cardiac causes of death, the major determinant of early post-resuscitation deaths.

In the absence of definitive data, severe hypotension and hypertension should be avoided, and mean arterial blood pressure should be targeted at achieving an adequate urinary output, taking into consideration the patient's pre-arrest blood pressure. Treatment using dobutamine has proved effective in supporting output and pressure during the post-resuscitation phase prior to return to baseline function.[26] Similarities in cardiovascular status between septic and post-resuscitation patients have indicated the 'early goal-directed therapy', which has proved effective in severe sepsis;[27] that is, normalization of intravascular volume, normalization of blood pressure by vasoactive drugs and normalization of oxygen transport by red cell transfusion during the first 6 hours post-resuscitation.[4,27] Data on its effectiveness in cardiac-arrest patients are not yet available.

### *Blood glucose*

A strong association between high blood glucose after resuscitation from cardiac arrest and poor neurologic outcome has been reported in several studies. Tight control of blood glucose (range 80–110 mg/dl or 4.4–6.1 mmol/l) with insulin reduces hospital mortality rates in critically ill adults;[28] in critically ill patients, the control of glucose level, with a target level of less than 8.0 mmol/l, rather than the dose of exogenous insulin, accounts for the improved survival,[29] but these findings have not been demonstrated specifically in cardiac-arrest patients.

In acute myocardial infarction (MI), the DIGAMI I study showed that the infusion of glucose and insulin followed by long-term insulin, improved long-term outcome among diabetic patients; this finding has not been confirmed by the DIGAMI II study, which identified elevated blood glucose as an independent predictor of adverse outcome. In conclusion, blood glucose post-ROSC should be monitored frequently, and hyperglycemia (above 6–8 mmol/l) should be treated with insulin infusion to avoid hypoglycemia.[30,31]

### *Acid–base status*

There is no randomized trial evaluating the possible benefit of treating acid–base disturbances. Acidosis has been demonstrated to be an adverse prognostic factor in the post-resuscitation phase: the washout of acid metabolites is completed shortly after restoration of spontaneous circulation, and persisting acidosis may indicate the continuing anaerobic metabolism, which has been described to result from the concurrence of failure of the heart to sustain circulation and altered peripheral oxygen utilization.[17]

In conclusion, the evidence for optimizing acid–base status is undetermined, but all interventions to avoid/correct severe acidosis appear reasonable.

### *Serum electrolytes*

No randomized trial has evaluated the value of changing serum potassium or magnesium in post-resuscitation care. However, hyperkalemia has been shown to be an adverse prognostic factor, although, from the existing data, it is impossible to determine whether the effect is per se or the result of acidosis or renal insufficiency. Hypomagnesemia is associated with adverse outcome in critically ill patients.

In conclusion, avoidance of hyperkalemia, hypokalemia and hypomagnesemia can be reasonably recommended, although without available evidence.

#### *Body temperature*

Evidence from several clinical studies suggests that hyperthermia/fever is commonly observed after cardiac arrest.[32,33] Hyperthermia/fever was identified as an independent risk factor associated with increased length of stay and higher mortality rate in a large, prospective study of patients admitted to a neurology/neurosurgical ICU.[34]

In comatose, post-arrest patients, each degree of body temperature over 37°C is associated with increased risk of unfavorable neurologic recovery,[35] and many of the benefits of mild therapeutic hypothermia may be related to the prevention of hyperthermia. In the comatose patient resuscitated from cardiac arrest, mild therapeutic hypothermia must be induced as soon and as fast as possible and maintained for 12–24 h post-ROSC (see below). If the patient is awake or if mild therapeutic hypothermia is contraindicated, any hyperthermia occurring in the first 72 h post-resuscitation should be promptly and aggressively treated with antipyretics or active cooling.

### Cardiac-oriented interventions

The most frequent cause of out-of-hospital cardiac arrest is cardiac[2] (presumed in 82.4% of cases). A treatment priority is to identify and treat the underlying cause of arrest, and this is particularly urgent in ischemic cardiac disease, which requires a time-dependent revascularization intervention. The high incidence of cardiac complications and fatal rearrest occurring in the first hours after ROSC strongly supports the stabilization of the patient and initiation of treatment to prevent the recurrence of arrest, including antiarrhythmic anti-ischemic treatment.

#### *Revascularization strategies*

Several postmortem studies have reported coronary atherosclerosis in 80% of cardiac arrests. Acute changes in coronary plaque morphology were described in 40–86% of cardiac-arrest survivors and in 15–64% at autopsy.[36,37] Immediate coronary angiography among survivors of out-of-hospital cardiac arrest showed coronary occlusion in 48% of cases, and this was not consistently associated with a corresponding ECG finding.[38]

In patients with cardiac arrest of presumed cardiac cause, thrombolytic treatment during CPR should be considered. After restoration of spontaneous circulation, the same rules as in acute coronary syndromes apply; that is, indication of the two revascularization techniques that are routine – thrombolysis and percutaneous transluminal coronary intervention – on the basis of characteristics and duration of symptoms, ECG findings and known contraindications.

The synthesis of consensus on science and available guidelines is reported below.

1. Thrombolysis
   - *Prehospital thrombolysis*: a meta-analysis of six trials involving 6434 patients reported a 17% decrease in mortality among patients treated with out-of hospital

fibrinolysis compared with in-hospital fibrinolysis.[39] The average time gained by out-of-hospital fibrinolysis was 60 min. Fibrinolytic therapy out-of-hospital to patients with ST elevation or signs and symptoms of acute coronary syndrome with presumed new left bundle branch block (LBBB) is beneficial. The efficacy is greatest within the first 3 h of the onset of symptoms.[39–42] (LOE 1).

In summary, out-of-hospital administration of fibrinolytics to patients with ST elevation myocardial infarction (STEMI) with no contraindications is safe, feasible and reasonable.

- *In-hospital thrombolysis* is recommended for patients with ST elevation (or presumably new LBBB) who have not received pre-hospital thrombolysis, if there are no facilities for immediate PCI.[43–47]

2. Percutaneous coronary intervention (PCI)
Coronary angioplasty with or without stent placement has become the first-line treatment for patients with ST elevation, because it has been shown to be superior to fibrinolysis in the combined endpoints of death, stroke and reinfarction in several studies and meta-analyses.[48–50]
   - Primary PCI is preferred in patients with symptom duration of over 3 h, if a skilled team can undertake it within 90 min after first patient contact, and in all patients with contraindications to fibrinolytic therapy. If the duration of symptoms is less than 3 h, the superiority of out-of-hospital fibrinolytic therapy, immediate in-hospital fibrinolytic therapy or transfer for primary PCI is not yet established clearly (class indeterminate).
   - Early revascularization (i.e., primary or facilitated PCI or surgery) is indicated for patients who develop shock within 36 h after symptom onset of acute myocardial infarction (AMI) and are suitable for revascularization.

*Anti-arrhythmic therapy*

- *Beta-blockade.* Several studies have shown that the administration of beta-blockers reduced total mortality (particularly sudden death), risk of recurrence and arrhythmia in patients with AMI and is associated with improved survival following resuscitation from cardiac arrest.[51–54] The indications for beta-blockers are known or recent myocardial infarction (MI) and cardiac arrest of presumed cardiac etiology, and they should be administered irrespective of the need of revascularization therapies.
- *Amiodarone.* Two large trials evaluating patients at risk of sudden death showed that amiodarone reduced arrhythmic deaths, but not total deaths. The indication for amiodarone is recurring ventricular arrhythmia, despite beta-blockade or if beta-blockade is not tolerated.[55,56]
- *Implantable cardioverter defibrillator (ICD).* The effectiveness of ICD therapy in both the primary and secondary prevention of SCD, has been analyzed. A meta-analysis of three trials comparing treatment with ICD to antiarrhythmics among in the patients with acute MI and depressed systolic myocardial function showed a significant reduction in death from any cause with ICD, with an average extended survival of 4 months in an observation period of 6 years, the benefit being greater in patients with a left ventricular ejection fraction of <35%. The balance of evidence favors ICD therapy over antiarrhythmic medical therapy in patients with previous SCD.[57]

## General ICU care

In the post-resuscitation phase, the patient requiring ICU is usually comatose and may not have regained spontaneous breathing. Besides the optimization of physiology, which may be obtained with more invasive methods and mild therapeutic hypothermia, such a patient requires ventilation and sedation.

### *Sedation*

Although there are no data to support or refute the use of a defined period of ventilation, sedation and neuromuscular blockade after cardiac arrest, it has been common practice to sedate and ventilate patients for up to 24h after ROSC. The duration of sedation and ventilation may be influenced by the use of therapeutic hypothermia (see below).

There are no data to indicate whether or not the choice of sedation influences outcome, but short-acting drugs (e.g., propofol, remifentanil, midazolam) will enable earlier neurologic assessment. An increased incidence of pneumonia has been reported when sedation is prolonged beyond 48h after pre-hospital or in-hospital cardiac arrest.[58]

In conclusion, sedation and analgesia may be beneficial immediately post-resuscitation and may be necessary to control shivering during hypothermia. If shivering continues despite optimal sedation, neuromuscular blockade may be required, but every attempt should be made to remove the sedatives/paralytics after the completion of hypothermia.

### *Ventilation*

Safar proposed maintaining $Pa_{O_2}$ over 100 mmHg and using minimal positive end-expiratory pressure (PEEP) after ROSC.[1,59] No data are available from human studies on the topic. The proposal to maintain $Pa_{O_2}$ over 100 mmHg and minimal PEEP for the first 24 h reflects common ICU practice.

Several studies in man and animals documented harmful effects of hypocapnia after cardiac arrest, but there are no data to support targeting of a specific $Pa_{CO_2}$ after resuscitation from cardiac arrest. Data extrapolated from patients with brain injury imply that ventilation to normocabia is appropriate.

Routine hyperventilation and the deriving hypocapnia during post-resuscitation ventilation of comatose survivors of cardiac arrest or brain trauma should be strictly avoided in order to prevent possible cerebral ischemia.

## Brain-oriented therapeutic interventions

### *Therapeutic hypothermia*

Mild therapeutic hypothermia is the only post-resuscitation intervention for which a clear-cut effect in improving neurologic outcome and survival has been demonstrated. Two randomized trials, published simultaneously in 2002, clearly demonstrated the beneficial effect of mild therapeutic hypothermia on outcome in comatose patients admitted to hospital after witnessed out-of-hospital ventricular fibrillation (VF) cardiac arrest.[60,61]

In the European[60] study (LOE 1), 275 patients resuscitated from witnessed VF of 15-min duration were randomized in nine centers to be treated with either normothermia (controls) or therapeutic hypothermia – 32–34°C bladder temperature induced and maintained by external cooling (a cool air-releasing blanket and mattress) for 24 h – and showed a significant improvement in favorable neurologic outcome at 6 months (Figure 9.2) and a significant decrease in 6-month mortality from 55% (controls) to 41% (cooled patients).

In the Australian study[61] (LOE 2), 77 patients, randomized in four centers to be treated with either normothermia or therapeutic hypothermia (33°C pulmonary artery temperature) induced and maintained by external cooling for 12 h, showed a significant improvement in neurologic outcome (Figure 9.2), although the difference in mortality rates between the normothermia group (68%) and the hypothermia group (51%) did not reach significance ($P = 0.145$).

A third trial took place in one of the centers also participating in the HACA study (LOE 2) on 30 comatose survivors of cardiac arrest with a primary ECG rhythm of asystole or pulseless electrical activity randomized to normothermia or hypothermia induced by external means and maintained for 4 h; they showed a significant improvement in metabolic endpoints that correlated with neurologic outcome.[62]

A recently published meta-analysis and systematic review[7] identified the previous studies as the only ones responding to the predefined requisites and analyzed the individual patient data provided by authors in a predefined set of variables, according to the intention-to-treat principle. More patients in the hypothermia group were discharged with favorable neurologic recovery (risk ratio, 1.68; 95% confidence interval, 1.29–2.07), and the number needed to treat to allow an additional patient to leave the hospital with favorable neurologic recovery was 6 (95% confidence interval 4–13).

In all the above studies, the induction and maintenance of hypothermia required prevention of shivering by adequate sedation, ventilation and neuromuscular blockade (bolus or continuous infusion) and no interference with coronary revascularization procedures. Rewarming at the end of the hypothermic period was performed slowly at a rate 0.25–0.5°C/h.[7,60–62]

Complications of mild therapeutic hypothermia have been reported to include increased infection, cardiovascular instability, coagulopathy, hyperglycemia and electrolyte abnormalities such as hypophosphatemia and hypomagnesemia.

However, in the meta-analysis, the use of mild therapeutic hypothermia showed no difference in the rate of occurrence of 'any complication'. Any bleeding occurred more often in the hypothermia group, but the difference was not statistically significant, despite the additive anticoagulation effects of hypothermia and those of coronary revascularization procedures. There was a trend toward a higher incidence of sepsis in the hypothermia group. Other complications such as pneumonia, renal failure and pancreatitis occurred equally in both groups.[7]

Based on this evidence, a dedicated advisory statement was published by the Advanced Life Support Task Force of ILCOR[63] recommending that:

- Unconscious adult patients with spontaneous circulation after out-of-hospital cardiac arrest should be cooled to 32–34 °C for 12–24 h when the initial rhythm was VF.
- Such cooling may also be beneficial for other rhythms or in-hospital cardiac arrest.

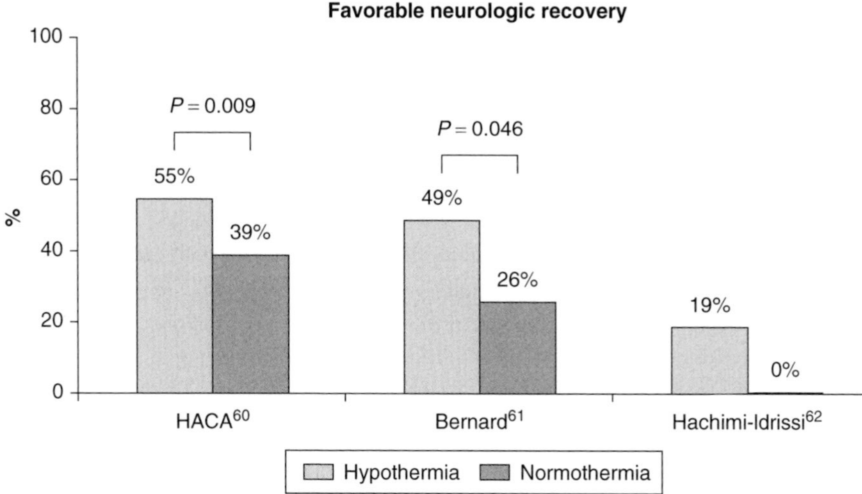


**Figure 9.2** Neurologic recovery in randomized trials of normothermia versus hypothermia induced by external means after resuscitation from cardiac arrest in patients. The Hachimi–Idrissi study analyzed metabolic endpoints that correlated to neurologic recovery.

The mechanism by which hypothermia is advocated to work is a multifactorial neuroprotective effect exerted during and after ischemic situations by simultaneously influencing several damaging pathways (see Madl & Holzer[64] for review).

Multiple studies in animals suggest that earlier and faster cooling after ROSC could significantly increase the potential benefit of hypothermia. Therefore, other techniques have been analyzed to improve the original cooling rate of 0.3°C/h obtained by external cooling such as the infusion of 30 ml/kg of 4°C saline to achieve a decrease in core temperature of approximately 1.5°C and intravascular cooling techniques to achieve a cooling rate of 1.5°C/h.[18–20]

Numerous other techniques are being developed, but further studies are needed to compare the effect of different cooling techniques on outcome and to identify optimum target temperature, rate of cooling, duration of hypothermia and rate of rewarming. In conclusion, mild therapeutic hypothermia should be started as soon as possible after resuscitation from cardiac arrest (with the most applicable technique) and maintained for 12–24 h. All patients comatose after out-of-hospital VF must be cooled, although hypothermia may be effective also after resuscitation from nonshockable rhythms and in-hospital arrest.

*Control of seizures*

Seizures or myoclonus occurs in 5–15% of adult patients who achieve ROSC, the rate rising to 40% if only comatose patients are considered.[65]

Seizures and myoclonus per se are not related significantly to outcome, but status epilepticus and, in particular, status myoclonus are associated with poor outcome.[66]

Seizures increase cerebral metabolism by up to fourfold and may precipitate life-threatening arrhythmia and respiratory arrest. For this reason, prompt and effective treatment of seizures is advocated, although the evidence is weak.

No studies have directly addressed the use of prophylactic anticonvulsant drugs after cardiac arrest in adults.[18–20] Anticonvulsants, such as thiopenthal and phenytoin, are neuroprotective, but a clinical trial of thiopenthal after cardiac arrest showed no benefit.[11] Further clinical studies are required.

In conclusion, the indication for anticonvulsants is undetermined, although their use in treatment of seizures is reasonable. Maintenance therapy should be started after the first event, once potential precipitating causes are excluded.[18–20]

### *Thrombolysis*

Thrombolytics, administered during arrest or early after reperfusion, have been shown in animal experiments to improve the microcirculation in the brain and may, by this mechanism, contribute to the favorable neurologic outcome of patients reported in many case reports and small case series with predominantly positive results.[67]

A multicenter, randomized trial on the effects of pre-hospital fibrinolysis on cerebral outcome is underway: the results, in terms of cerebral bleeding, are especially relevant, in view of the indication for pre-hospital fibrinolysis for coronary revascularization.

*In summary, to optimize cerebral recovery besides moderate hypothermia it is important to maintain adequate blood pressure, to control oxygenation, glycemia and acidosis and to treat seizures (see above).*

## PROGNOSTIC EVALUATION

After restoration of spontaneous circulation, the organ that influences most significantly both survival and the quality of survival is the brain. Possible outcomes range from complete neurologic recovery to death to persistent vegetative state. Of the patients initially resuscitated from cardiac arrest and admitted to ICU, almost 80% remain comatose for varying lengths of time, 40% remain in a vegetative state, and up to 80% are dead at 1 year.[64] Even in selected patients with witnessed cardiac arrest after VF and cardiac arrest with advanced life support no longer than 15 min, the mortality rate at 6 months is 45–55%.[60]

The period after resuscitation can be extremely stressful to the families of patients because their questions about the patient's ultimate prognosis cannot be answered conclusively. Ideally, a clinical assessment, laboratory test or biochemical marker able to predict outcome in the acute setting, either during cardiac arrest or immediately after resuscitation, could help provide sound information to families and contribute to reduce the possibility of less than optimal cerebral outcome. Such a test of prognosis should have a specificity of 100%.

Although research has been conducted in man and animals on the predictive value of neurologic signs and biochemical markers during cardiac arrest and in the first hours after ROSC, the studies are not conclusive, and the ILCOR consensus on science concludes that relying on neurologic examination or biochemical markers during the acute phase to predict outcome is not recommended and should not be used.[18]

The value of early prediction of neurologic outcome has been brought into question by the evidence that post-reperfusion complex secondary post-reflow cerebral derangements lead to impaired cerebral reperfusion and death of vulnerable neurons, with further deterioration of cerebral outcome[63] (for review, see Madl & Holzer[64]), which does not become definitive until 24 h post-resuscitation.

To monitor the evolution of the depth of coma and prognosticate outcome in the first days after resuscitation, a variety of methods have been proposed, including neurologic examination, electrophysiologic techniques and biochemical tests.

The physical examination, which should include separate recording of the three components of the Glasgow Coma Scale (GCS) – best motor response, best verbal response and eye opening spontaneously and to standardized verbal and painful stimulation – and of the brainstem reflex evaluation, has the potential to be extremely useful in the common clinical scenario because of its universal availability and ease of performance.

A recent meta-analysis[68] reviewed the reliability of single signs at different time intervals post-resuscitation in 11 studies involving almost 200 patients. Five clinical signs were found strongly to predict death or poor neurologic outcome, with four of the five predictors detectable at 24 h post-resuscitation:

- absent corneal reflex at 24 h
- absent pupillary response at 24 h
- absent withdrawal response to pain at 24 h
- no motor response at 24 h
- no motor response at 72 h.

A systematic review identified the recording of somatosensory evoked potentials (SSEP) as the method with the highest prognostic validity.[69]

The predictive value of SSEP acquired in the first 3 days after resuscitation was studied in a meta-analysis, reviewing 18 studies in 1136 patients with post-hypoxic ischemic encephalopathy: the results showed that normothermic adults in coma after cardiac arrest with no cortical SSEP response have a chance of awakening of less than 1%.[70]

Routine use of the ECG is not supported by the results of the published reviews, except when seizure activity is suspected.[70] However, the finding of grades I (normal alpha with theta delta activity), IV (alpha coma, spikes, sharp waves, slow waves with very little background activity) and V (very flat to isoelectric) on EEGs performed in comatose patients at least 24–48 h after cardiac arrest, can support the prediction of unfavorable outcome.[18]

Serum levels of molecular markers for brain injury have been studied with respect to the detection of the extent of cerebral damage and neurologic outcome in cardiac-arrest survivors. In particular, increased serum levels of the neuron-specific enolase (NSE), a cytoplasmic enzyme of glycolysis, and the astroglial protein S100, a calcium-binding protein regulating neuronal differentiation and apoptosis, are known to be associated with hypoxic–ischemic brain injury and unfavorable neurologic outcome.[71]

A recent study tested the value of serial serum NSE (measured at admission and daily post-insult) in combination with GCS and SSEP to predict neurologic prognosis in unconscious patients admitted to the ICU after resuscitation from cardiac arrest. High serum NSE levels in comatose patients at 24 and 48 h after CPR predict poor neurologic outcome. Addition of NSE to GCS and SSEP increases predictability.[72]

## CONCLUSION

In conclusion, to improve the outcome of patients resuscitated from cardiac arrest, an aggressive and focused therapeutic approach is mandatory. Strong evidence supports time-dependent therapeutic interventions, which should be performed as early as possible after restoration of spontaneous circulation, i.e. coronary reperfusion, beta blockade and hypothermia in the comatose patient. Mild therapeutic hypothermia, initiated as early as possible and maintained for 24 h, improves neurologic outcome and survival of one patient in every six treated and does not interfere with coronary reperfusion interventions. After initiation of hypothermia, the care of the comatose patient post-resuscitation should focus on optimizing physiology and maintaining brain-oriented care, always remembering that cerebral damage may worsen in the post-resuscitation phase if physiology is not optimized. Prognosis can be reliably formulated at 24–72 h post-resuscitation, and aggressive intensive care should be maintained at least until a reliable prognostic evaluation can be formulated.

## REFERENCES

1. Safar P, Behringer W, Böttiger BW et al. Cerebral resuscitation potentials for cardiac arrest. Crit Care Med 2002; 30(Suppl): 140–4.
2. Pell JP, Sirel JM, Marsden AK et al. Presentation, management, and outcome of out of hospital cardiopulmonary arrest: comparison by underlying aetiology. Heart 2003; 89: 839–42.
3. Cummins RO, Ornato JP, Thies WH, Pepe PE. Improving survival from sudden cardiac arrest: the 'chain of survival' concept. A statement for health professionals from the Advanced Cardiac Life Support Subcommittee and the Emergency Cardiac Care Committee, American Heart Association. Circulation 1991; 83(5): 1832–47.
4. Adrie C, Laurent I, Monchi M et al. Post-resuscitation disease after cardiac arrest: a sepsis-like syndrome? Curr Opin Crit Care 2004 ; 10(3): 208–12.
5. Langhelle A, Tyvold SS, Lexow K et al. In-hospital factors associated with improved outcome after out-of-hospital cardiac arrest. A comparison between four regions in Norway. Resuscitation 2003; 56: 247–63.
6. Skrifvars MB, Rosenberg PH, Finne P et al. Evaluation of the in-hospital Utstein template in cardiopulmonary resuscitation in secondary hospitals. Resuscitation 2003; 56: 275–82.
7. Holzer M, Bernard SA, Hachimi-Idrissi S et al. Hypothermia for neuroprotection after cardiac arrest: systematic review and individual patient data meta-analysis. Crit Care Med 2005; 33(2): 414–18.
8. Rea TD, Eisenberg MS, Sinibaldi G, White RD. Incidence of EMS-treated out-of-hospital cardiac arrest in the United States. Resuscitation 2004; 63: 17–24.
9. Parish DC, Dane FC, Montgomery M et al. Resuscitation in the hospital: relationship of year and rhythm to outcome. Resuscitation 2000; 47(3): 219–29.
10. Peberdy MA, Kaye W, Ornato JP et al. Cardiopulmonary resuscitation of adults in the hospital: a report of 14 720 cardiac arrests from the National Registry of Cardiopulmonary Resuscitation. Resuscitation 2003; 58: 297–308.
11. Cerchiari EL, Ferrante M. Postresuscitation syndrome. In: Paradis NA, Halperin HR, Novak RM, eds. Cardiac Arrest. The Science and Practice of Resuscitation Medicine. Baltimore: Williams and Wilkins, 1996: 837–949.
12. Brain Resuscitation Clinical Trial I Study Group. Randomized clinical study of thiopental loading in comatose survivors of cardiac arrest. N Engl J Med 1986; 314: 397–403.
13. Becker LB, Ostrander MP, Barrett J et al. Outcome of cardiopulmonary resuscitation in a large metropolitan area: where are the survivors? Ann Emerg Med 1991; 20: 355–61.
14. Negovsky VA, Gurvitch AM, Zolo-tokrylina ES. Post Resuscitation Disease. Amsterdam: Elsevier, 1983.
15. Engdahl J, Holmberg M, Karlson BW, Luepker R, Herlitz J. The epidemiology of out-of-hospital 'sudden' cardiac arrest. Resuscitation 2002; 52(3): 235–45.
16. Ebell MH, Becker LA, Barry HC, Hagen M. Survival after in-hospital cardiopulmonary resuscitation. A meta-analysis. J Gen Intern Med 1998; 13(12): 805–6.

17. Laurent I, Monchi M, Chiche JD et al. Myocardial dysfunction after cardiac arrest. J AM Coll Cardiol 2002; 40(12): 2110–6.
18. International Liaison Committee on Resuscitation. IV. Advanced life support. Resuscitation 2005; 67: 213–47
19. European Resuscitation Guidelines. Resuscitation 2005; Suppl 1.67: 213–47
20. Herlitz J, Castren M, Friberg H et al. Post resuscitation care. What are the therapeutic alternatives and what do we know? Resuscitation 2006; 69(1): 15–22.
21. Bell DB, Brindley PG, Forrest D et al. Management following resuscitation from cardiac arrest: recomendations from the 2003 Rocky Mountain Critical Care Conference. Can J Anaesth 2005; 52(3): 309–22.
22. Mullner M, Domanovits H, Sterz F et al. Measurement of myocardial contractility following successful resuscitation: quantitated left ventricular systolic function utilising noninvasive wall stress analysis. Resuscitation 1998; 39: 51–9.
23. Cerchiari EL, Safar P, Klein E, Cantadore R, Pinsky M. Cardiovascular function and neurologic outcome after cardiac arrest in dogs: the cardiovascular post-resuscitation syndrome. Resuscitation 1993; 25: 9–33.
24. Kern KB, Hilwig RW, Rhee KH, Berg RA. Myocardial dysfunction after resuscitation from cardiac arrest: an example of global myocardial stunning. J Am Coll Cardiol 1996; 28: 232–40.
25. Tang W, Weil MH, Sun S et al. Epinephrine increases the severity of postresuscitation myocardial dysfunction. Circulation 1995; 92: 3089–93.
26. Tennyson H, Kern KB, Hilwig RW, Berg RA, Ewy GA. Treatment of post resuscitation myocardial dysfunction: aortic counterpulsation versus dobutamine. Resuscitation 2002; 54: 69–75.
27. Rivers E, Nguyen B, Havstad S et al. Early goal-directed therapy in the treatment of severe sepsis and septic shock. N Engl J Med 2001; 345: 1368–77.
28. van den Berghe G, Wouters P, Weekers F et al. Intensive insulin therapy in the critically ill patients. N Engl J Med 2001; 345: 1359–67.
29. Finney SJ, Zekveld C, Elia A, Evanse TW. Glucose control and mortality in critically ill patients. JAMA 2003; 290: 2041–7.
30. Malmberg K, Ryden L, Efendic S et al. Randomized trial of insulin-glucose infusion followed by subcutaneous insulin treatment in diabetic patients with acute myocardial infarction (DIGAMI Study). Effects on mortality at 1 year. J Am Coll Cardiol 1995; 26: 57–65.
31. Malmberg K, Ryden L, Wedel H et al for the DIGAMI 2 investigators. Intense metabolic control by means of insulin in patients with diabetes mellitus and acute myocardial infarction (DIGAMI 2): effects on mortality and morbidity. Eur Heart J 2005; 26: 650–61.
32. Takino M, Okada Y. Hyperthermia following cardiopulmonary resuscitation. Intensive Care Med 1991; 17: 419–20.
33. Takasu A, Saitoh D, Kaneko N, Sakamoto T, Okada Y. Hyperthermia: is it an ominous sign after cardiac arrest? Resuscitation 2001; 49: 273–7.
34. Diringer MN, Reaven NL, Funk SE, Uman GC. Elevated body temperature independently contributes to increased length of stay in neurologic intensive care unit patients. Crit Care Med 2004; 32: 1489–95.
35. Zeiner A, Holzer M, Sterz F et al. Hyperthermia after cardiac arrest is associated with an unfavorable neurologic outcome. Arch Intern Med 2001; 161: 2007–12.
36. Davies MJ, Thomas A. Thrombosis and acute coronary-artery lesions in sudden cardiac ischemic death. N Engl J Med 1984; 310: 1137–40.
37. Zipes DP, Wellens HJJ. Sudden cardiac death. Circulation 1998; 98: 2334–51.
38. Spaulding CM, Joly L-M, Rosenberg A et al. Immediate coronary angiography in survivors of out-of-hospital cardiac arrest. N Engl J Med 1997; 336: 1629–33.
39. Morrison LJ, Verbeek PR, McDonald AC, Sawadsky BV, Cook DJ. Mortality and prehospital thrombolysis for acute myocardial infarction: a meta-analysis. JAMA 2000; 283: 2686–92.
40. Welsh RC, Goldstein P, Adgey J et al. Variations in prehospital fibrinolysis process of care: insights from the assessment of the safety and efficacy of a new thrombolytic 3 plus international acute myocardial infarction pre-hospital care survey. Eur J Emerg Med 2004; 11: 134–40.

41. Weaver W, Cerqueira M, Hallstrom A et al. Prehospital initiated vs hospital-initiated thrombolytic therapy: the Myocardial Infarction Triage and Intervention Trial (MITI). JAMA 1993; 270: 1203–10.
42. European Myocardial Infarction Project Group (EMIP). Prehospital thrombolytic therapy in patients with suspected acute myocardial infarction. The European Myocardial Infarction Project Group. N Engl J Med 1993; 329: 383–9.
43. Indications for fibrinolytic therapy in suspected acute myocardial infarction: collaborative overview of early mortality and major morbidity results from all randomised trials of more than 1000 patients. Fibrinolytic Therapy Trialists' (FTT) Collaborative Group. Lancet 1994; 343: 311–22.
44. Effectiveness of intravenous thrombolytic treatment in acute myocardial infarction. Gruppo Italiano per lo Studio della Streptochinasi nell'Infarto Miocardico (GISSI). Lancet 1986; 1: 397–402.
45. The GUSTO investigators. An international randomized trial comparing four thrombolytic strategies for acute myocardial infarction. N Engl J Med 1993; 329: 673–82.
46. Boersma E, Maas AC, Deckers JW, Simoons ML. Early thrombolytic treatment in acute myocardial infarction: reappraisal of the golden hour. Lancet 1996; 348: 771–5.
47. De Luca G, van't Hof AW, de Boer MJ et al. Time-to-treatment significantly affects the extent of ST-segment resolution and myocardial blush in patients with acute myocardial infarction treated by primary angioplasty. Eur Heart J 2004; 25: 1009–13.
48. Weaver WD, Simes RJ, Betriu A et al. Comparison of primary coronary angioplasty and intravenous thrombolytic therapy for acute myocardial infarction: a quantitative review. JAMA 1997; 278: 2093–8.
49. Keeley EC, Boura JA, Grines CL. Primary angioplasty versus intravenous thrombolytic therapy for acute myocardial infarction: a quantitative review of 23 randomised trials. Lancet 2003; 361: 13–20.
50. Widimsky P, Budesinsky T, Vorac D et al. Long distance transport for primary angioplasty vs immediate thrombolysis in acute myocardial infarction. Final results of the randomized national multicentre trial—PRAGUE-2. Eur Heart J 2003; 24: 94–104.
51. The MIAMI Trial Research Group. Metoprolol in acute myocardial infarction (MIAMI): a randomised placebo-controlled international trial. Eur Heart J 1985; 6: 199–226.
52. Randomised trial of intravenous atenolol among 16 027 cases of suspected acute myocardial infarction: ISIS-1. First International Study of Infarct Survival Collaborative Group. Lancet 1986; 2: 57–66.
53. Halkin A, Grines CL, Cox DA et al. Impact of intravenous beta-blockade before primary angioplasty on survival in patients undergoing mechanical reperfusion therapy for acute myocardial infarction. J Am Coll Cardiol 2004; 43: 1780–7.
54. Yusuf S, Peto R, Lewis J, Collins R, Sleight P. Beta blockade during and after myocardial infarction: an overview of the randomized trials. Prog Cardiovasc Dis 1985; 27: 335–71.
55. Cairns JA, Connolly SJ, Roberts R, Gent M, for the Canadian Amiodarone Myocardial infarction Arrhythmia Trial Investigators. Randomised trial of outcome after myocardial infarction in patients with frequent or repetitive ventricular premature depolarisations: CAMIAT. Lancet 1997; 349: 675–82.
56. Julian DG, Camm AJ, Frangin G et al. Randomised trial of effect of amiodarone on mortality in patients with left ventricular dysfunction after recent myocardial infarction: EMIAT. European Myocardial Infarct Amiodarone Trial Investigators. Lancet 1997; 349: 667–74.
57. Connolly SJ, Hallstrom AP, Cappato R et al. Meta-analysis of the Implantable cardioverter defibrillator secondary prevention trials. AVID, CASH and CIDS studies. Antiarrhythmics vs Implantable Defibrillator study. Cardiac Arrest Study Hamburg. Canadian Implantable Defibrillator Study. Eur Heart J 2000; 21: 2071–8.
58. Rello J, Valles J, Jubert P et al. Lower respiratory tract infections following cardiac arrest and cardiopulmonary resuscitation. Clin Infect Dis 1995; 21: 310–4.
59. Safar P. Cerebral resuscitation after cardiac arrest: a review. Circulation 1986; 74(6 Pt 2): IV-138–53.

60. The Hypothermia after Cardiac Arrest study group. Mild therapeutic hypothermia to improve the neurologic outcome after cardiac arrest. N Engl J Med 2002; 346: 549–56.
61. Bernard SA, Gray TW, Buist MD et al. Treatment of comatose survivors of out-of-hospital cardiac arrest with induced hypothermia. N Engl J Med 2002; 346: 557–63.
62. Hachimi-Idrissi S, Corne L, Ebinger G, Michotte Y, Huyghens L. Mild hypothermia induced by a helmet device: a clinical feasibility study. Resuscitation 2001; 51(3): 275–81.
63. Nolan JP, Morley PT, Hoek V, Hickey RW. Therapeutic hypothermia after cardiac arrest. An advisory statement of the Advanced Life Support Task Force of the International Liaison Committee on Resuscitation. Circulation 2003; 108: 118–21.
64. Madl C, Holzer M. Brain function after resuscitation from cardiac arrest. Curr Opin Crit Care 2004; 10(3): 213–7.
65. Krumholz A, Stern BJ, Weiss HD. Outcome from coma after cardiopulmonary resuscitation: relation to seizures and myoclonus. Neurology 1988; 38: 401–5.
66. Wijdicks EF, Parisi JE, Sharbrough FW. Prognostic value of myoclonus status in comatose survivors of cardiac arrest. Ann Neurol 1994; 35: 239–43.
67. Böttiger BW, Bode C, Kern S et al. Efficacy and safety of thrombolytic therapy after initially unsuccessful cardiopulmonary resuscitation: a prospective clinical trial. Lancet 2001; 357: 1583–5.
68. Booth CM, Boone RH, Tomlinson G, Detsky AS. Is this patient dead, vegetative, or severely neurologically impaired? Assessing outcome for comatose survivors of cardiac arrest. JAMA 2004; 291: 870–9.
69. Zandbergen EG, de Haan RJ, Stoutenbeek CP, Koelman JH, Hijdra A. Systematic review of early prediction of poor outcome in anoxic-ischaemic coma. Lancet 1998; 352: 1808–12.
70. Robinson LR, Micklesen PJ, Tirschwell DL et al. Predictive value of somatosensory evoked potentials for awakening from coma. Crit Care Med 2003, 31: 960–7.
71. Snyder-Ramos SA, Gruhlke T, Bauer H et al. Cerebral and extracerebral release of protein S100B in cardiac surgical patients. Anaesthesia 2004; 59(4): 344–9.
72. Meynaar IA, Straaten HM, van der Wetering J et al. Serum neuron-specific enolase predicts outcome in post-anoxic coma: a prospective cohort study. Intensive Care Med 2003; 29: 189–95.

# 10

# Sudden death in children and adolescents

Nicola Carano and Umberto Squarcia

Sudden death describes unexpected natural death within a short period of time, generally less than 1 h from the onset of symptoms, or unwitnessed death during sleep in a person without any prior condition that would appear fatal.[1] This excludes death from violent or accidental causes. Pediatric sudden unexpected natural death involves infants, children and adolescents; fortunately, it is rare. Population-based reports show specific rates of 1.3–8.0 per year per 100 000 inhabitants.[2–5]

Because the subject of this volume is sudden cardiac death (SCD) but noncardiac sudden death in the pediatric age group has a relatively high rate, it is necessary to review briefly noncardiac causes of pediatric sudden death.

In infancy, many sudden deaths are caused by sudden infant death syndrome (SIDS), which is defined as 'the sudden death of an infant under one year of age which remains unexplained after a thorough case investigation, including performance of a complete autopsy, examination of the death scene and review of the clinical history'.[6] SIDS is still an enigma in infantile pathology, and since it is a distinct topic from sudden death in children and adolescents, it will not be considered in this chapter. Not all infants who die suddenly have SIDS: other infant-specific causes of sudden death under 1 year of age are infections, some unrecognized congenital heart diseases (particularly duct-dependent heart malformation and severe obstructive anomalies in the systemic circulation), primary arrhythmia, complete congenital atrioventricular block and intracranial hemorrhage.

## NONCARDIAC SUDDEN DEATH IN CHILDREN AND ADOLESCENTS

Sudden death may be attributed either to known pre-existing diseases or to causes discovered at autopsy. In some cases, the sudden death remains unexplained even after necropsy. The report by Wren et al showed a 23% cardiovascular cause in the group with a previously known disease. The percentage of cardiovascular causes rose to 30% when the death was caused by an abnormality discovered at autopsy. These data indicate that many other causes of sudden death occur in children and adolescents.[5] They are listed in Table 10.1.

Sudden death from asthma affects 1/10 000 asthmatic children.[7] In spite of the increased knowledge of the pathogenesis and progresses in therapy, it continues to occur.[8] In asthmatic children, sudden death results from hypoxia due to sudden and severe onset of airway closure.

| **Table 10.1** Noncardiac causes of sudden death |
|---|
| Asthma |
| Epilepsy |
| Infections |
| • Fulminant bronchopneumonia |
| • Epiglottitis |
| • Meningitis |
| • Septic shock |
| Pulmonary embolism |
| Intracranial hemorrhage |
| Cerebral edema |
| Acute hydrocephalus |

Sudden death may also be caused by epilepsy, particularly in patients with severe disease, poor control and poor compliance with drugs.[9,10] Apnea and hypoxia secondary to seizures, cardiac arrhythmia, and drug overdose or drug withdrawal are the mechanisms that have been proposed. In some instances, the diagnosis of epilepsy as the cause of sudden death may be wrong: in fact, primary cardiac arrhythmia may cause syncope and anoxic seizures, leading to a wrong diagnosis.[11] In the study by Wren et al, asthma and epilepsy, respectively, were the causes of sudden death in the 21% and 34% of cases in which death was attributed to a known pre-existing condition.[5] Infections accounted for the 57% in the group in which the cause was discovered at autopsy.[5]

Unexpected and sudden death from infectious causes frequently occurs after slight symptoms of an apparently trivial disease of short duration in healthy individuals (inflammation of the upper respiratory tract, fever, sore throat, fatigue, and headache).

Causes of sudden death also include known unexpected complications of disease of which the patient is at risk. A typical example of this situation is pulmonary embolism, which is rare in the pediatric age group.[12] Predisposing factors include congenital heart disease, sepsis, arteriovenous malformations, prolonged immobility, in-dwelling venous catheters, malignancy (neoplastic embolism), and hypercoagulative states.

Cerebral edema may be caused by head trauma, syndrome of inappropriate antidiuretic hormone or by diabetic ketoacidosis. The onset may be rapid and the condition may lead to sudden death.

Sudden death may also be due to intracranial hemorrhage. It may occur as result of rapid bleeding into one or more of the intracranial compartments, such as the extradural, subdural, subarachnoid, and intraventricular spaces, or into brain tissue. In children and adolescents, intracranial hemorrhage with the potential for sudden death is caused by a rupture of vascular lesions, as in cavernous hemangioma, arteriovenous malformation and arterial aneurysm. The last one is frequently associated with coarctation of the aorta, polycystic kidney disease, and Ehlers–Danlos syndrome.

Severe coagulation disorder such as hemophilia or other coagulation factor deficiencies, thrombocytopenic inherited purpura, and afibrinogenemia are potential causes of intracranial hemorrhage.

In acute obstructive hydrocephalus, an intracranial lesion in a crucial site adjacent to a ventricular foramen acutely obstructs the free flow of cerebrospinal fluid. Acute hydrocephalus usually is caused by a lesion in the posterior fossa. At the Hospital for Sick Children in Toronto, in a 4-year period, acute obstructive hydrocephalus caused sudden death in seven patients with previously undiagnosed intracranial tumor.[13]

## SCD IN INFANTS AND ADOLESCENTS

In retrospective studies that focus on SCD in people aged 1–22 years, the incidence of sudden death from cardiac causes is 1.3–4.6 per 100 000 patients per year.[2–4] In apparently normal children beyond the first year of life, the incidence of sudden death is probably around 1–1.5 per 100 000 per year.[5] This is in contrast to the much higher incidence of SCD in adults, which is reported to be 1/1000 population per year. Thus, SCD in children and adolescents is rare, but recent studies suggest that its incidence is increasing.[14] Because many cases of SCD occur during sports activities, another source of data is the National Center for Catastrophic Sport Injury Research, an organization that collects reports of serious injury and death during competitions by high-school and college athletes in the USA. From data reported in 2000 by this organization, a total annual incidence of one case per 350 000 high-school athletes per year can be estimated.[15]

Table 10.2 lists the causes of SCD in children and adolescents. The causes are classified into five subdivisions as follows: coronary artery abnormalities, myocardial abnormalities, operated and unoperated congenital heart diseases, primary arrhythmia and other conditions. Many of the causes of SCD are familial.

### Coronary artery abnormalities

Isolated congenital coronary artery anomalies may entail a significant risk of myocardial ischemia, myocardial dysfunction, congestive heart failure and sudden death. Conventionally, imaging of coronary arteries has been done with selective coronary angiography. More recently, magnetic resonance imaging (MRI) has also been used, but the continuous improvements in ultrasound technology have made delineation of coronary artery anatomy feasible in many children and adolescents.[16] Therefore, the evaluation of coronary anatomy by transthoracic echocardiography has become an integral part of the evaluation of patients with cardiac symptoms such as exercise-induced chest pain and syncope.[16]

#### *Anomalous origin of a coronary artery from the opposite sinus of Valsalva*

This anomaly has been associated with myocardial ischemia, ventricular arrhythmia and sudden death,[17–20] particularly when the anomalous coronary artery courses between the great arteries. In anomalous origin of the left coronary artery from the right sinus of Valsalva, the left main coronary artery arises from the right aortic sinus and passes between the aorta and the pulmonary artery before dividing into the left anterior descending and left circumflex arteries. In anomalous origin of the right coronary artery from the left sinus of Valsalva (Figure 10.1), the right coronary artery arises from the left aortic sinus and passes between the aorta and the pulmonary artery before its usual distribution.

The anomalously originating coronary artery may be intramyocardial if it courses within the myocardial sulcus between the great arteries, or intramural if it courses in

**Table 10.2** Causes of sudden cardiac death in children and adolescents

| |
|---|
| **Coronary artery abnormalities** |
| Left coronary artery arising from pulmonary artery |
| Right coronary artery arising from pulmonary artery |
| Left coronary artery arising from the right sinus of Valsalva |
| Right coronary artery arising from the left sinus of Valsalva |
| Single coronary artery ostium |
| Coronary ostial stenosis in Williams syndrome |
| Coronary aneurysm in Kawasaki disease |
| **Myocardial abnormalities** |
| Hypertrophic cardiomyopathy* |
| Dilated cardiomyopathy* |
| Restrictive cardiomyopathy |
| Arrhythmogenic right ventricular dysplasia* |
| Myocarditis |
| **Operated and unoperated congenital heart diseases** |
| Aortic valve stenosis |
| Tetralogy of Fallot |
| Transposition of the great arteries |
| Aortic dissection (coarctation of the aorta and Marfan's syndrome*) |
| Ebstein's anomaly |
| Fontan operation |
| ***Primary arrhythmia*** |
| Channelopathy |
| Long-QT syndrome* |
| Brugada syndrome* |
| Andersen syndrome* |
| Catecholaminergic polymorphic ventricular tachycardia* |
| Wolf–Parkinson–White syndrome |
| Heart block |
| ***Other conditions*** |
| Pulmonary hypertension |
| Commotio cordis |
| Drug abuse |
| Anorexia nervosa |
| Cardiac tumor |

*May be familial.

the anterior aortic wall between the great arteries. Three mechanisms have been proposed to explain myocardial ischemia in the anomalously originating coronary artery:

1. The ostium of the anomalously originating coronary artery is slit-shaped, and this can compromise coronary reserve (Figure 10.1B).
2. The anomalously originating coronary artery usually arises from the aorta not perpendicularly but at an acute angle, and this can alter the flow into arteries (Figure 10.1B).
3. The interarterial course puts the anomalously originating coronary artery at risk of compression between the great arteries. This theory seems unlikely because the pulmonary artery pressure is low in normal individuals even during exercise. Rather than being due to the compression, myocardial ischemia is probably due

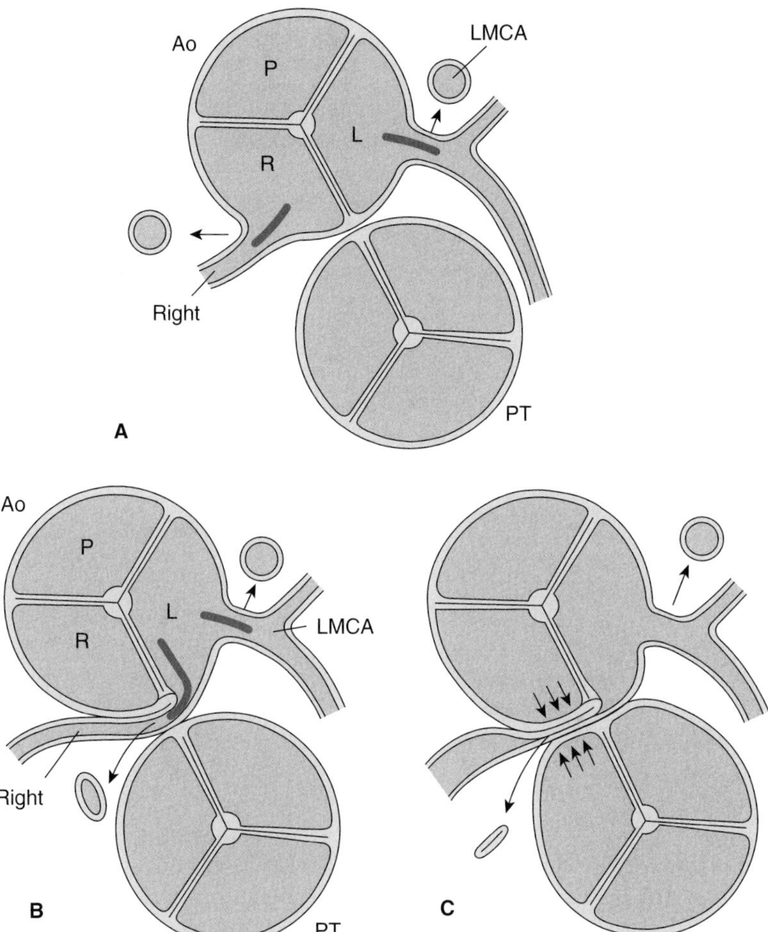


**Figure 10.1** (A) Diagrammatic representation of the normal origin of the coronary arteries from the appropriate sinus of Valsalva. (B) Anomalous origin of the right coronary artery from the left coronary sinus, with interarterial course. The ostium is slit-shaped, and the right coronary artery arises with an acute angle. This can alter the flow into the artery. (C) When aortic wall tension increases with exercise, the right coronary artery becomes flattened. As a consequence, the flow is reduced and ischemia can occur. Ao = aorta; PT = pulmonary trunk; right = right coronary artery; LMCA = left main coronary artery; P = posterior (noncoronaric) sinus of Valsalva; R = right sinus of Valsalva; L = left sinus of Valsalva; Arrows = cross-area of coronary arteries.

to deformation of the anomalous intramural coronary artery when aortic pressure and aortic wall tension increase during exercise. In fact, the wall tension is determined by the radius of the vessel, so the aorta will have greater wall tension than the intramural coronary artery, and the anomalous coronary artery will become flattened when aortic wall tension increases. Therefore, coronary artery flow will be reduced as long as the myocardial oxygen supply is inadequate (Figure 10.1C).

The left coronary artery from the right sinus with interarterial course has an estimated incidence of 0.03–0.05%[21] but is frequently associated with SCD[17] that usually occurs with exercise. Sudden death from this anomaly particularly affects young people during or shortly after high-intensity exercise.[18] Fifty percent of patients who died suddenly were asymptomatic without a previous episode of chest pain, syncope, palpitations or diagnosed arrhythmia. In the series reported by Barth & Roberts, all the 23 patients who were younger than 20 years of age died suddenly during or just after exercise.[18]

The anomalous right coronary artery from the left sinus has an incidence of 0.1%.[21] It is associated with sudden death: 13 of the 52 patients reported by Taylor et al died suddenly (six deaths were exercise-related) and the victims were previously asymptomatic.[22] Therefore, data from the literature suggest that anomalous origin of either coronary artery from the opposite sinus with an interarterial course carries a significant risk of SCD, particularly in young athletes, and that symptoms frequently are absent before death.[18,22] When symptoms are present, they are related to myocardial ischemia. In a recent review by Frommelt et al, 10 children and adolescents were prospectively identified as carriers of anomalous origin of coronary artery from the opposite sinus with an interarterial course.[23] Of the 10 patients (with age ranging from 3 months to 20 years), four underwent cardiac evaluation because of exercise-induced syncope, chest pain or ventricular tachycardia, and the other six had transthoracic echocardiography for suspected congenital heart disease. All four symptomatic patients were participating in vigorous physical activity when symptoms developed: this suggests that strenuous exercise is the trigger for myocardial ischemia in this condition. Sudden death is rare before adolescence, but in cases with associated coronary ostial stenosis at the origin of the anomalous coronary artery, sudden death has been reported also in infants and children.[24,25] Clinical examination, ECG and chest radiography are not helpful in diagnosing the anomalous origin of the coronary artery because ischemia and myocardial dysfunction do not occur at rest. A normal exercise test does not ensure that the patient is risk free. Transthoracic echocardiography has become an important noninvasive tool to identify the anomalous origin of the coronary artery from the opposite sinus. Identification of the anomaly requires focused two-dimensional echocardiography and color Doppler imaging of the coronary artery.[16,23] Coronary angiography, ultrafast computed tomography (CT) and MRI may be necessary to clarify the anatomy of the coronary artery. Symptomatic patients with anomalous origin of the coronary artery require surgical correction. Many surgical techniques have been used, including coronary bypass, patch enlargement of the anomalous coronary origin, reimplantation of the anomalous coronary artery in the appropriate sinus, and unroofing of the intramural segment. Early results with the unroofing technique seems to be promising.[23] The unroofing procedure is increasingly used even in asymptomatic children electively after the age of 10 because the risk of sudden death before adolescence seems to be low.[26]

### *Single coronary artery*

About 43% of cases of this anomaly are associated with other cardiac malformations (transposition of the great arteries, tetralogy of Fallot, and truncus arterosus). The single coronary artery can arise from either the right or the left sinus of Valsalva.

Most cases of single coronary artery produce no symptoms, but small numbers of premature death have been reported in those variants in which a major branch passes between the aorta and the pulmonary artery.[27]

*Anomalous origin of the left coronary artery from the pulmonary artery*

Anomalous origin of the left coronary artery from the pulmonary artery is a rare congenital anomaly in which the left coronary artery arises from the pulmonary trunk, and then courses adjacent to its normal aortic origin before branching into the left circumflex and left anterior descending artery. After birth, when pulmonary vascular resistance falls, the intercoronaric anastomosis provides communication between a high-resistance vessel (the aorta and the right coronary artery) and a low-resistance vessel (the pulmonary artery and the left coronary artery). This determines a pressure gradient in the coronary circle with the flow from the aorta to the pulmonary artery through the right coronary artery, the intercoronaric anastomosis and the left coronary artery. The perfusion of the left coronary artery is retrograde, and a steal of blood in the coronary bed occurs. The time of presentation, during childhood, is variable and is related to the adequacy of collateral circulation between the right and the left coronary arteries. On the basis of myocardial ischemia, symptomatic infants present with clinical signs of congestive heart failure and echocardiographic signs of severely dilated cardiomyopathy. They may die from congestive heart failure or suddenly from ventricular arrhythmia.

Patients who are diagnosed later in childhood often are asymptomatic and usually present a murmur or cardiomegaly on chest radiography. Their late presentation is due to efficient collateral circulation that partially preserves left ventricular function. Ischemic injury still occurs and results in papillary muscle fibrosis, mitral regurgitation and progressive left ventricular dilation. Sudden death with exercise has been described and is probably due to limited coronary reserve with development of ventricular arrhythmia when myocardial demand increases. The anomalous origin of the left coronary artery from the pulmonary artery may be identified by echocardiography, which provides direct visualization of the insertion of the left coronary artery into the pulmonary trunk, significant right coronary artery dilation, abnormal diastolic flow signal within the ventricular septum, retrograde filling of the left coronary artery and abnormal diastolic flow in the pulmonary artery, as the anomalous left coronary artery empties into the pulmonary artery. Echocardiographic findings of left ventricular dysfunction and mitral valve regurgitation coexist. So all children with echocardiographic findings suggestive of dilated cardiomyopathy should be evaluated for the origin of the coronary arteries. ECG findings may suggests anterolateral myocardial infarction. Cardiac catheterization and selective coronary angiography are the definitive confirmation test. Surgical treatment actually consists of implantation of the anomalous coronary artery into the aorta, or the creation of an intrapulmonary tunnel that connects the aorta with the anomalous coronary artery. Late complications after surgery include occlusion or stenosis of the reimplanted coronary artery, reduced myocardial reserve and chronic mitral valve dysfunction.

*Anomalous origin of the right coronary artery from the pulmonary artery*

Unlike the anomalous origin of the left coronary artery from the pulmonary artery, the anomalous origin of the right coronary artery from the pulmonary artery is asymptomatic in the great majority of patients. However, syncope, cardiac arrest, sudden death and angina pectoris (due to coronary steal) have been described.[28] There may be a continuous murmur at the left sternal border. The anomaly can be recognized by echocardiographic color Doppler and coronary angiography.

*Coronary ostial stenosis*

This anomaly has been reported also in infants.[29] Patients may present with sudden death, angina pectoris, myocardial infarction or congestive heart failure. Coronary ostial stenosis is rare and usually occurs in patients with Williams syndrome, a complex syndrome comprising developmental abnormalities, craniofacial dysmorphic features, and cardiac anomalies, typically supravalvular aortic stenosis and multiple peripheral pulmonary artery stenosis. Williams syndrome is related to the deletion of the elastine gene located in chromosome 7. Coronary ostium may be involved in the supravalvular aortic stenosis, and this can determine the stenosis,[30] but severe coronary ostial stenosis has been described also in the absence of supravalvular aortic stenosis.[31]

*Coronary abnormalities in Kawasaki disease*

Kawasaki disease occurs mostly in young children (80% of patients are younger than 4 years). In Kawasaki disease, there is vasculitis of the coronary artery with dilation of coronary arteries and possible formation of aneurysms. Because of thrombotic occlusion and stenotic obstruction, coronary aneurysms may cause myocardial infarction and death. Furthermore, coronary artery vasculitis and the consequent intimal hypertrophy may impair myocardial flow reserve and endothelial function.[32] Thus, after Kawasaki disease, even in the late follow-up, potential causes of myocardial ischemia and sudden death may exist. Patients who have chronic coronary artery abnormalities may need anticoagulation therapy. Activity restriction and periodical evaluation of myocardial perfusion by thallium perfusion scan, dobutamine stress echocardiography and selective coronary angiography may be necessary. Coronary bypass is indicated for patients with significant myocardial ischemia.

## Myocardial abnormalities

Dilated cardiomyopathy and especially hypertrophic cardiomyopathy are important causes of sudden death. The structural abnormalities involve fibrosis and cellular hypertrophy with resultant cellular architectural disarray. These structural abnormalities provide an electrical substrate for re-entrant arrhythmia. Cellular and architectural changes also provide a dyshomogeneous electrical substrate with resultant arrhythmia. Another possible substrate for sudden death in myocardial abnormality is ischemia. Especially in hypertrophic cardiomyopathy, there may be small coronary artery disease secondary to medial hypertrophy. The resultant ischemia can determine arrhythmia by re-entrant or automatic mechanism.

*Hypertrophic cardiomyopathy*

Hypertrophic cardiomyopathy is characterized by left ventricular and/or right ventricular hypertrophy that can be asymmetric and affect different regions of the ventricle. Ventricular cavities are usually normal or small in size. Systolic intraventricular gradients are common. Microscopically, an extensive disarray of hypertrophied myocardial cells, myocardial scarring and abnormalities of small intramural coronary arteries is present. Familial disease with autosomal dominant inheritance predominates. The clinical course varies markedly: some patients remain asymptomatic throughout life, others have symptoms of heart failure, and others die suddenly, often in the absence of previous symptoms. Symptomatic patients who die suddenly have usually presented anginal chest pain and syncope on exercise. They are prone to develop arrhythmia that leads to sudden death.[33] In a study of 99 children with hypertrophic cardiomyopathy in Toronto, the reported annual combined risk of sudden death and cardiac arrest was 2.7% at 8–18 year of age.[34] In this study, the occurrence of syncope did not predict sudden death, whereas ventricular tachycardia on ambulatory ECG recording was a significant risk factor for this. As sudden death occurs during or shortly after exercise, affected children should avoid sports or intense physical exercise. Sudden death from previously unrecognized hypertrophic cardiomyopathy is rare, with an age-specific risk in apparently normal children or adolescents of less than 1:1 000 000 per year.[5,35] A necropsy diagnosis of hypertrophic cardiomyopathy should lead to screening for other family members, but, because of variable penetrance or because the new case represents a new mutation, no other cases may be found. The first gene for familial hypertrophic cardiomyopathy was mapped to chromosome 14q11.2–q12. Soon thereafter, familial locus heterogeneity was reported by mapping of other loci.[36] All the disease-causing genes encode proteins that are part of a sarcomere. Studies in the genotype–phenotype relation are providing the evidence that the prognosis for patients who have different mutations varies considerably.[36] In patients who are considered at risk of life-threatening tachyarrhythmia, the available therapeutic options for the prevention of sudden death are medical treatment with amiodarone and the implantable cardioverter defibrillator (ICD).

### *Dilated cardiomyopathy*

Sudden death in dilated cardiomyopathy is uncommon, congestive heart failure being the most frequent cause of death. Friedmann et al reported one sudden death in a series of 63 children in a period of 10 years.[37] Muller et al reported four sudden deaths in a series of 28 children during a mean follow-up of 4.1 years.[38] Sudden death in dilated cardiomyopathy is due to ventricular tachycardia or ventricular fibrillation. Electrophysiologically guided therapy and implantable defibrillators may have a role in the treatment of patients with malignant tachyarrhythmia.

### *Restrictive cardiomyopathy*

Restrictive cardiomyopathy has a high mortality in children. Rivenes et al reported 64.7% mortality in a series of 18 patients during a mean follow-up of 2.6 years. Sudden death occurred in 28% of the patients in this series.[39] Patients who died suddenly were apparently well and had no evidence of heart failure, but they often had signs or symptoms of ischemia manifested clinically by chest pain, syncope or both.

### *Arrhythmogenic right ventricle dysplasia*

Arrhythmogenic right ventricle dysplasia is a myocardial disease that typically affects the right ventricle: it is characterized histologically by the gradual replacement of myocites by adipose and fibrous tissue.[40] The disorder is an important cause of sudden death in people under 30 years of age; 80% of cases are diagnosed between the ages of 15 and 40 years.[40] The anatomic substrate of arrhythmogenic right ventricle dysplasia can result in right ventricular tachyarrhythmia and sudden death. Clinically, arrhythmogenic right ventricle dysplasia presents in young men with syncope, ventricular tachycardia of left-bundle branch block morphology, cardiac arrest or, rarely, congestive heart failure. On the ECG, it is common to find T-wave inversion in V1–V3 and ε waves, which are small post-excitation electrical potentials that occur at the end of the QRS complex and at the beginning of the ST segment. In addition, MRI is used to diagnose arrhythmogenic right ventricle dysplasia. Arrhythmogenic right ventricle dysplasia is inherited as an autosomal dominant trait with variable penetrance and incomplete expression. Genetic heterogeneity (eight loci) has been identified for this autosomal dominant form.[36] Treatment strategies include beta-blockers, amiodarone, radiofrequency ablation and intracardiac cardioverter-defibrillators.

*Myocarditis*

Myocarditis severe enough to be recognized clinically is rare, but the prevalence of mild and subclinical cases is probably much higher. Myocarditis is most often due to Coxsackievirus and ECHO virus, but many other viruses can cause it. Cardiac involvement is unpredictable and may involve the conduction system, causing heart block, or the myocardium, causing depression of ventricular function and/or ventricular tachyarrhythmia. These can lead to sudden death. The majority of patients, especially those with only mild inflammation, recover completely. Some patients experience persistent cardiomegaly, with or without signs of congestive heart failure, and are indistinguishable from those with dilated cardiomyopathy. The management may include anticongestive therapy, ventricular pacing and antiarrhythmic drugs. Rest and avoidance of exertion are important during the acute and healing phases and until the echocardiographic findings, ambulatory ECG monitoring and exercise testing return to normal.

## Operated and unoperated congenital heart diseases

Two old studies described the most common cause of sudden death in patients with known structural heart disease.[41,42] Since those two reports, the management strategies have changed, and surgical and interventional techniques and intensive care abilities have improved, but, in spite of that, sudden death still remains a significant problem for some unoperated and operated cardiovascular diseases. In a variety of congenital heart disease, tachyarrhythmia and bradyarrhythmia are common mechanisms involved in the sudden death events.[43] The electrical substrate underlying the development of arrhythmia involves fibrosis and hypertrophy of cardiac chambers, and fibrosis of conduction cardiac tissue. These changes are secondary to the hemodynamic stress in the native lesion or to the surgical repair in the operated lesion. Changes in myocardial tissue can lead to re-entry circuit or abnormal automaticity. Therefore, the substrate for arrhythmia in the patient with native aortic stenosis is hypertrophy, whereas in the patient who had surgical repair of tetralogy of Fallot, the scar caused from surgery may become the substrate for tachyarrhythmia or bradyarrhythmia.

*Aortic valve stenosis*

Older children and young adults who have significant unoperated aortic valve stenosis or significant residual stenosis after either surgical commissurotomy or balloon valvuloplasty are at risk of exercise-related sudden death. The valve obstruction leads to increased wall stress, compensatory left ventricular hypertrophy and increased myocardial oxygen demands. During exercise, when the systemic and myocardial demands are high, the coronary blood flow, which is primarily a diastolic event, may not sufficiently increase because of inadequate augmentation of cardiac output, due to valve stenosis, and because of tachycardia, decreased systemic vascular resistance and decreased diastolic blood pressure induced by exercise, which reduce diastolic perfusion. These phenomena can compromise myocardial oxygen supply and lead to cellular ischemia, which may cause malignant dysrhythmia and sudden death. When aortic regurgitation coexists, myocardial ischemia on exercise may be even more severe because aortic insufficiency further reduces diastolic perfusion pressures and increases left ventricular end-diastolic pressure. The incidence of sudden death in children with aortic stenosis is 4–20%.[44]

The presence of serious arrhythmia, multiform premature ventricular contraction, ventricular couplets and ventricular tachycardia has been associated with male sex, higher left ventricle end-diastolic pressure, aortic regurgitation and high probability of sudden death.[45]

*Tetralogy of Fallot*

Tetralogy of Fallot consists of the association between a large ventricular septal defect and an obstruction of the right ventricle outflow tract, with the aorta overriding the ventricular septal defect. Depending on the severity of the right ventricle outflow tract obstruction, the direction and the magnitude of the shunt through the ventricular septal defect vary. With severe stenosis, the shunt is right to left, the pulmonary blood flow is decreased and cyanosis appears. Infants and children who have unoperated tetralogy of Fallot may suffer from hypoxic spells that usually occur in the morning and are characterized by restlessness and prolonged crying, increased cyanosis, hyperpnea and decreasing intensity of the murmur. These spells may lead to syncope, seizures or sudden death.

Patients with tetralogy of Fallot that have undergone reparative surgery have a 4.6–6% risk of sudden death between 3 months and 20 years of age.[43,46] Sudden death occurs particularly in patients who have residual defects (ventricular septal defect, significant pulmonary stenosis, or significant pulmonary regurgitation), increased right ventricular pressure and ventricular arrhythmia. Ventricular arrhythmia is present in about 50% of the patients, occurring particularly in patients who were older at the time of surgery or in patients with significant pulmonary regurgitation, ventricular dysfunction and duration of QRS of more than 180 ms. Hemodynamic and electrophysiologic sequelae of surgical repair of tetralogy of Fallot could decrease with earlier operative repair, improved bypass techniques and limitation of pulmonary regurgitation by adequate transannular patch or valved conduits. Correction of significant residual hemodynamic abnormalities is important to reduce the incidence of sudden death in such patients.

### *Complete transposition of the great arteries*

In complete transposition of the great arteries, there is a ventriculoarterial discordance due to an abnormal septation of the fetal conotruncus: the aorta arises from the right ventricle, and the pulmonary artery from the left. This anomaly results in the recirculation of the deoxygenated systemic venous blood in the aorta and in the recirculation of oxygenated pulmonary venous blood in the pulmonary arteries. Neonates with complete transposition of the great arteries are at risk of death when sufficient mixing of systemic and pulmonary circulation does not occur across an atrial septal defect or a ventricular septal defect. Therefore, neonates with insufficient mixing need balloon atrioseptostomy in the first hours of life.

The atrial switch operation for complete transposition of the great arteries (Figure 10.2) has a progressive risk of atrial arrhythmia. About two-thirds of patients suffer from arrhythmia after a mean follow-up of 18 years.[47] These patients tend to lose sinus rhythm gradually and suffer from supraventricular tachycardia, junctional rhythm, atrial flutter, ventricular tachycardia and atrioventricular block. Anatomic substrates for arrhythmia in atrial switch patients are related to extensive resection necessary in the area of the atrial conduction tissue, with resultant fibrosis, and with progressive dilation and dysfunction of the systemic right ventricle. With normal atrioventricular node conduction, the ability of very rapid conduction to the ventricles exists; therefore, the mechanism of SCD is thought to be atrial tachyarrhythmia, usually atrial flutter, with rapid conduction to ventricles.[47–49] The impaired right ventricular function, which usually is present in these patients, reduces tolerance of the tachyarrhythmia.[48] Because the Mustard and Senning operation is no longer performed, the incidence of SCD in patients having had repair for transposition will decline.

### *Congenitally corrected transposition of the great arteries*

Congenitally corrected transposition of the great arteries is characterized by atrioventricular and ventriculoarterial discordance. Patients with this anomaly are predisposed to spontaneous development of atrioventricular block. Because of associated anomalies and unpredictable substitutive pacemaker activity, sudden heart block may not be well tolerated and may lead to sudden death.

### *Aortic dissection*

Aortic dissection occurs in patients who have systemic hypertension and inheritable disorder of connective tissue such as Marfan's syndrome or Ehlers–Danlos syndrome. Aortic dissection may present also in children. The genetic abnormality of Marfan's syndrome has been localized to fibrillin genes of chromosome 15. In Marfan's syndrome, the walls of major arteries show microscopic medial disruption and disorganization, which predispose to aortic dissection. Prompt attention to chest pain and assessment of aortic size with ultrasound, CT or MRI are advised in Marfan's syndrome. Long-term administration of beta-blockers seems to decrease the likelihood of aortic complication in Marfan's syndrome. Patients with unrepaired or repaired coarctation are also at risk of aortic dissection. In the aorta, adjacent to the coarctation site, changes of cystic medial necrosis commonly occur. This may provide a histologic substrate for late aneurysm formation or aortic dissection. All patients who have coarctation are at increased risk of developing systemic hypertension. Moreover, even patients with mild resting gradient and a good operative repair may be at risk of developing significant exercise-induced hypertension.

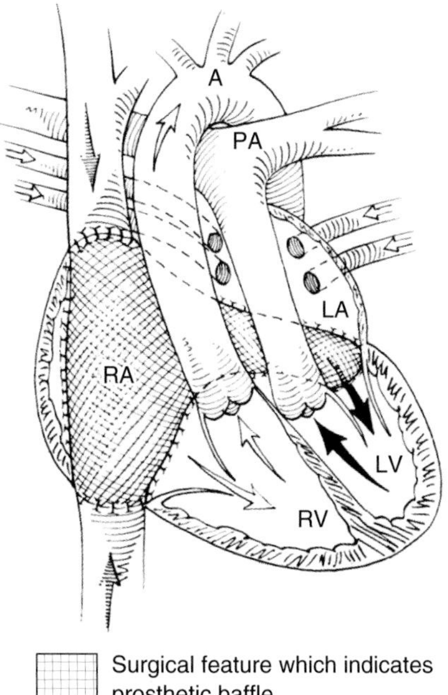


**Figure 10.2** Diagrammatic representation of the Mustard and Senning operation in complete transposition of the great arteries. A pericardial or prosthetic baffle is placed in the atria (the atrial septum has been excised) in such a way as to redirect the pulmonary venous blood to the right atrium and the systemic venous blood to the left atrium. With this kind of atrial switch operation, the pulmonary and the systemic circulations are in series, but the right ventricle continues to support the systemic circulation. RA = right atrium; LA = left atrium; RV = right ventricle; LV = left ventricle; PA = pulmonary artery; A = aorta.

*Ebstein's anomaly*

In Ebstein's anomaly, tricuspid valve leaflets are displaced toward the apex of the right ventricle. The anomaly causes variable degrees of tricuspid insufficiency and limitation of forward flow. Ebstein's anomaly often is associated with the presence of accessory atrioventricular conduction pathways, which may be evident or not on standard ECG. Celermajer et al reported five sudden deaths in their series of 50 neonates with Ebstein's anomaly (average age at death was 4.5 years).[50]

Sudden death in patients with Ebstein's anomaly is due in most cases to atrial fibrillation (caused by atrial enlargement from tricuspid regurgitation) with very rapid ventricular response through an accessory atrioventricular pathway, leading to ventricular tachycardia or ventricular fibrillation.

*The Fontan operation*

The Fontan operation is performed in a great variety of complex congenital heart diseases with a single functioning ventricle. The aim of this operation is to separate the pulmonary circulation from the systemic in single-ventricle congenital heart disease. This is obtained by creating a connection between the caval veins, the right atrium and the pulmonary artery, so that the whole systemic venous return flows toward the lungs. For many years, the Fontan operation was performed by creating an anastomosis between the right atrium and the pulmonary artery trunk (Figure 10.3A). Sinus node dysfunction and atrial tachyarrhythmia are common after this type of surgery; the most likely substrate is the extensive atrial resection with consequent scarring and fibrosis. This anatomic substrate can be potentiated by hemodynamic factors such as higher systemic venous pressure and the resulting right atrium dilation. Sudden death can occur: it is thought to be caused by atrial tachyarrhythmia, mainly atrial flutter with rapid conduction to the ventricle through the atrioventricular node. Recent studies suggest that deranged cardiac autonomic nervous activity may also have an important role in the late arrhythmogenesis of Fontan patients.[51] Therapy includes antiarrhythmic drugs, antitachycardia pacing, and radiofrequency ablation.[52] The modified Fontan operation, mainly total cavopulmonary connections (by intracardiac tunnel or extracardiac conduit) reduces surgical involvement of the right atrium and eliminates the influence of the increased systemic venous pressure on the right atrial wall. This new surgical technique (Figure 10.3B) seems to reduce or eliminate the life-threatening atrial arrhythmia. For this reason, older Fontan patients who have a direct anastomosis between the right atrium and the pulmonary artery are being converted to the extracardiac total cavopulmonary connection.

## Primary arrhythmia

The great majority of SCD that remain unexplained even after necropsy are probably due to primary cardiac arrhythmia. Types of arrhythmia that may be fatal and that do not leave traces after death include cardiac channelopathy, a class of heritable arrhythmic syndromes that are due to defective ion channels in the heart and present with syncope, seizures and sudden death. These include the long-QT syndrome (LQTS), Brugada syndrome, catecholaminergic polymorphic ventricular tachycardia and Andersen syndrome. Other kinds of potentially fatal primary arrhythmia not caused by channelopathy include atrial fibrillation in Wolff–Parkinson–White syndrome and congenital complete atrioventricular block.

### *The long-QT syndrome (LQTS)*

LQTS is an inherited or acquired disorder of repolarization that is identified by the ECG abnormality of prolongation of QT interval (QT corrected for the heart rate by Bazett's formula) greater than 460 ms.[53] Other ECG abnormalities in LQTS are relative bradycardia, T-wave abnormalities (broad-based, biphasic, bifid or notched, and alternans T wave) and episodic ventricular tachycardia, particularly torsade de pointes. During these episodes, cardiac output is markedly impaired, and this can result in syncope, but torsade de pointes has the potential to degenerate into ventricular fibrillation, leading to sudden death.

LQTS may be either congenital or acquired. Romano–Ward syndrome is the most common congenital form and is transmitted as an autosomal dominant trait. Jervell and Lange-Nielsen syndrome is the uncommon inherited form; it is transmitted as an autosomal recessive trait and is associated with neurosensorial deafness. Patients with the last variant have a more severe course and higher rates of sudden death.[54] There are many causes of acquired LQTS; medication is the most common (Table 10.3). Acquired LQTS usually presents later in life.

Congenital LQTS most commonly presents during childhood and adolescence with recurrent episodes of syncope,[55] which are precipitated by intense emotion,

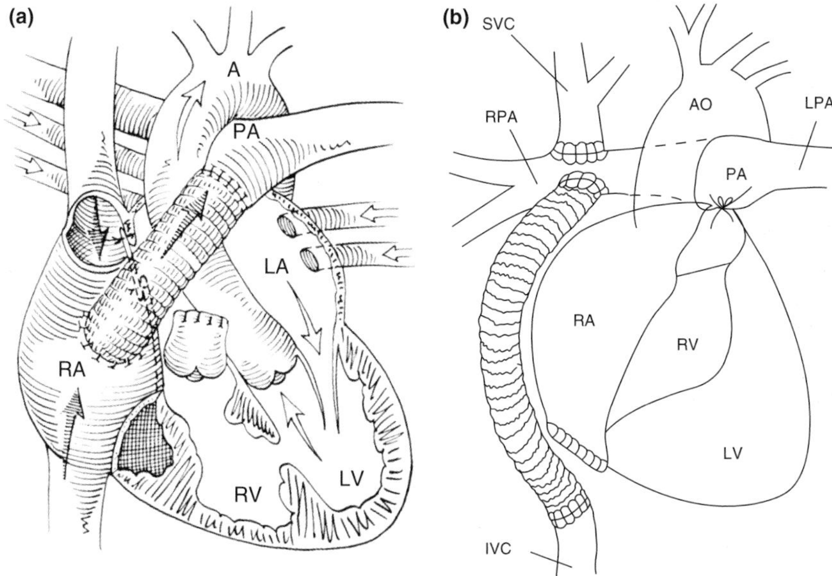


**Figure 10.3** (a) Diagrammatic representation of one of the oldest modifications of the Fontan operation. A prosthetic conduit connects the right atrium with the pulmonary artery. The proximal pulmonary artery has been sutured. With this operation, the whole systemic venous return goes to the lungs, bypassing the right ventricle. The right atrial progressive dilation occurring with this type of circulation, together with the extensive surgical involvement of the atrial wall, is the anatomic substrate for tachyarrhythmia in the long-term follow-up. RA = right atrium, LA = left atrium; RV = right ventricle, LV = left ventricle, PA = pulmonary artery, A = aorta, striped arrows indicate blood flow from right atrium to pulmonary artery through the conduit. (b) The most modern modification of the Fontan operation: the extracardiac total cavopulmonary connection. The systemic venous blood goes to the lungs via a bidirectional Glenn anastomosis (superior vena cava to right pulmonary artery) and across an extracardiac conduit from the inferior vena cava to the right pulmonary artery. The right atrium is much less involved in the surgery. This technique seems to reduce or eliminate late atrial tachyarrhythmia. SVC and IVC = superior and inferior vena cava; LPA and RPA = left and right pulmonary arteries; PA = pulmonary artery; AO = aorta; RA = right atrium; RV = right ventricle; LV = left ventricle striped section indicates extra cardiac conduit.

vigorous physical activities and loud noises (alarm clock or ringing telephone). Approximately 10% of children with LQTS will present sudden death.[55]

Approximately two-thirds of LQTS are secondary to mutation that involves six genes that encode the primary or auxiliary subunits of the cardiac channel: *KCNQ1* (LQT1), *KCNH2* (LQT2), *SCN5A* (LQT3), *ANK2* (LQT4), *KNE1* (LQT5) and *QKCNE2* (LQT6).[55] Molecular genetic methods showed that a cutoff value of ≥460 ms was most appropriate in identifying definitively gene carriers.[53] The therapy of LQTS aims to reduce the sympathetic activity of the heart either pharmacologically or surgically. Beta-blockers are the initial therapy of choice; propranolol (2–4 mg/kg per day, maximum 60 mg/day) and nadolol (0.5–1 mg/kg per day, maximum 2.5 mg/day) are the most commonly used. In patients refractory to this treatment, left-sided cervicothoracic sympathetic ganglionectomy has been shown to be effective.[55] For patients who continue to be symptomatic despite treatment, implantation of a cardioverter-defibrillator is indicated.

**Table 10.3** Causes of acquired long-QT syndrome

| |
|---|
| **Cardiac** |
| Complete heart block, severe bradycardia |
| Coronary artery disease |
| Myocarditis |
| **Metabolic** |
| Alcoholism |
| Anorexia nervosa |
| Electrolyte abnormalities (hypocalcemia, hypokalemia, hypomagnesemia) |
| Hypothyroidism |
| **Neurologic** |
| Cerebrovascular accident |
| Encephalitis |
| Subarachnoid hemorrhage |
| Traumatic brain injury |
| **Drugs** |
| Antidysrhythmics (classes 1A and 3) |
| Antiemetic (droperidol) |
| Antifungal (ketoconazole) |
| Antihistamines (astemizole, terfenadine) |
| Antimicrobials (erythromycin, trimetoprim-sulfamehoxazole) |
| Antipsychotics (haloperidol, risperidone) |
| Organophosphate insecticides |
| Phenothiazines (thioridazine) |
| Promotility agents (cisapride) |
| Tricyclic antidepressants (amitriptyline) |

*Andersen syndrome*

The phenotype of Andersen syndrome includes hypokalemic periodic paralysis, dysmorphic features, QTc prolongation and polymorphic ventricular tachycardia. The dysmorphic features include syndactyly, hypertelorism, low-set ears, broad forehead, micrognathia, cleft palate and scoliosis.[56] Andersen syndrome is inherited as an autosomal dominant trait. Mutation of the gene *KCNJ2* accounts for nearly half of the cases.

*Brugada syndrome*

Brugada syndrome describes the association of polymorphic ventricular tachycardia and ventricular fibrillation with a typical ECG pattern of right-bundle branch block with ST elevation in leads V1–V3 at rest or during provocation with sodium calcium blockers (ajmaline or procainamide).[57] Brugada syndrome can present with SCD, particularly at night. Mutation in the cardiac sodium channel that is encoded by the gene *SCN5A* provides the pathogenetic molecular substrate for Brugada syndrome, but accounts for only 10–20% of cases.[58]

*Catecholaminergic polymorphic ventricular tachycardia*

This disorder is characterized by the occurrence of bidirectional and polymorphic ventricular tachycardia in relation to adrenergic stimulation of physical activity, but without evidence of structural myocardial disease and without QT prolongation.[59]

The clinical outcome of these patients is poor, with estimates of mortality at 30–50% by the age of 20–30 years.[59] Children frequently present with syncope or seizures. As in the other channelopathies, patients can be misdiagnosed with epilepsy. Mutations in the cardiac ryanodine receptors, which are encoded by *RYR2* (*CPVT1*), and calsequestrin, which is encoded by *CASQ2* (*CPVT2*), have been identified.[60]

Currently, the implantable cardioverter-defibrillator represents the frontline therapy for patients with channelopathy at risk of lethal arrhythmia.

### *Wolff–Parkinson–White syndrome*

Wolff–Parkinson–White syndrome is one of the most common causes of supraventricular tachycardia in children, but sudden deaths are rare. Sudden death is due to ventricular fibrillation, which is precipitated by atrial fibrillation in patients with a short anterograde accessory pathway refractory period.[61] The combination of Wolff–Parkinson–White syndrome and atrial fibrillation is very unusual in children. Catheter ablation of the accessory pathway is indicated in patients with previous cardiac arrest or syncope.

### *Congenital complete atrioventricular block*

Congenital complete atrioventricular block without associated heart disease affects about one baby in every 20 000. It can frequently be associated with maternal collagen disease. Nearly all cases are recognized at birth or in early infancy. If the heart is structurally normal, bradycardia is relatively well tolerated; however, during long-term follow-up, some patients develop Adam–Stokes attacks and sudden death. The risk of sudden death is related to the ventricular rate and to the concomitance of ventricular arrhythmia (bradycardia-related, QT prolongation and torsade de pointes). Pacemaker implantation is indicated in patients who are symptomatic or have congestive heart failure.

## Other conditions

### *Pulmonary hypertension*

Secondary pulmonary hypertension (pulmonary vascular obstructive disease) usually occurs as a consequence of some congenital heart disease such as large ventricular septal defect, large ductus arteriosus, complete atrioventricular canal, truncus arteriosus or total anomalous pulmonary venous drainage. Pulmonary vascular obstructive disease is the result of elevated pulmonary artery pressure and increased pulmonary blood flow and occurs when congenital heart diseases that are associated with large left to right shunt and pulmonary hypertension undergo delayed correction or are not repaired. Pulmonary hypertension and increased pulmonary blood flow lead to progressive pulmonary artery damage that includes medial hypertrophy, extension of smooth muscle into nonmuscular arterioles, intimal hyperplasia, occlusion, fibrosis and arteritis. The arterial damage is believed to occur more frequently and more quickly in children with Down's syndrome. Arterial damage increases pulmonary vascular resistance, limiting pulmonary blood flow and progressively reversing the shunt, which becomes right to left, resulting in progressive cyanosis (Eisenmenger's syndrome). Patients become progressively exercise limited and can die suddenly with or without a triggering stimulus such as exertion, cold inspired air or coughing. Sudden death is rare in children and adolescents, but it becomes progressively more frequent in the third decade of life. The mechanism of sudden death is believed to be secondary to acute pulmonary hypertensive crisis with increasing hypoxia or dysrhythmia. Other noncardiac causes of sudden death in Eisenmenger's syndrome are intrapulmonary hemorrhage, stroke and thromboembolism. Because of the early repair of congenital heart disease, Eisenmenger's syndrome has become rare.

Pulmonary hypertension is defined as primary when all other causes of pulmonary hypertension are excluded. Primary pulmonary hypertension is rarely diagnosed in children and may be familial. Anatomic lesions in the pulmonary arteries are similar to those seen in the secondary type. In the presence of markedly elevated pulmonary vascular resistance, the right ventricle becomes unable to maintain normal function, and the resting cardiac output decreases. The symptoms include dyspnea on exertion, chest pain and syncope. Syncope is often exertional or post-exercise and implies severely restricted output, leading to diminished cerebral blood flow that may be further impaired by peripheral vasodilation during exercise. The natural course in primary pulmonary hypertension is more rapid than in secondary forms. Before the era of vasodilator therapy (calcium channel blockers, continuous IV prostacyclin, nitric oxide, and bosentan), most children died, sometimes suddenly, within 1 year of the diagnosis.

### *Commotio cordis*

Commotio cordis is life-threatening dysrhythmia caused by a direct, nonpenetrating blow to the chest. It is characterized by sudden disturbance of the cardiac rhythm in the absence of demonstrable signs of mechanical injury to the heart.[62] Commotio cordis is most commonly limited to the sudden onset of ventricular fibrillation, but may be manifested as other cardiac rhythm disturbances such as heart block, ventricular tachycardia, bundle block, ST-wave changes or asystole. Using a swine model, Link et al found that ventricular fibrillation could be produced by an impact applied in a window of vulnerability that occurred 30–15 ms before the peak of the T wave.[63] Commotio cordis has been described in baseball and ice-hockey players who undergo chest trauma and in victims of child abuse.

### *Drug abuse*

Cocaine causes vasoconstriction, myocardial ischemia and ventricular tachyarrhythmia, and simultaneously increases the heart rate and blood pressure. Sudden death can occur independently of the amount, prior use or route of administration, and regardless of underlying heart disease.[64]

### *Anorexia nervosa*

There is a risk of sudden death in patients with anorexia nervosa because of an imbalance of electrolytes, extreme bradycardia and prolonged QT interval.[65]

### *Cardiac tumors*

It is uncommon for sudden death to occur as the result of undiagnosed cardiac tumor.[66] The most common cardiac tumors in the pediatric age group are rhabdomyoma and cardiac fibroma, but atrial myxoma has also been observed. Syncope and sudden death can result from acute hemodynamic disturbance in the form of obstruction of ventricular inflow or outflow, or from lethal tachyarrhythmia or sudden atrioventricular block.

## SUMMARY

This chapter has reviewed the potential causes of sudden death in children and adolescents. Many patients who die suddenly have identifiable cardiac disease and are known to have been at risk; however, other cardiac conditions, such as hypertrophic cardiomyopathy or primary arrhythmia such as LQTS, may not be known. Many patients who have hypertrophic cardiomyopathy, primary arrhythmia or LQTS, but who do not have symptoms, can be screened with careful and detailed personal and family history. Worrisome features that demand careful investigation includes syncope during or immediately after exercise and a family history of premature sudden death or of life-threatening events. Any patients with positive familial and personal history should receive an ECG and echocardiography, which can detect most, not all, of the diseases that may lead to sudden death in children and adolescents.

## REFERENCES


1. Myerburg RJ. Sudden cardiac death: epidemiology, causes and mechanisms. Cardiology 1997; 74: 2–9.
2. Molander N. Sudden natural death in later childhood and adolescents. Arch Dis Child 1982; 57: 572–6.
3. Driscoll DJ, Edwards WD. Sudden unexpected death in children and adolescents. J Am Coll Cardiol 1985; 5: 118B–21B.
4. Neuspiel DR, Kuller LH. Sudden and unexpected natural death in childhood and adolescence. JAMA 1985; 254: 1321–5.
5. Wren C, O'Sullivan JJ, Wright C. Sudden death in children and adolescents. Heart 2000; 83: 410–3.
6. Byard RW, Krous HF. Sudden infant death syndrome: overview and update. Perspect Pediatric Pathol 2003; 6: 112–27.
7. Champ CS, Byard RW. Sudden death in asthma in childhood. Forensic Sci 1984; 66: 117–27.
8. Strunk RC. Death due to asthma. Am Rev Respir Dis 1993; 148: 550–2.
9. Nashef L, Sander JW. Sudden unexpected death in epilepsy. Where are we now? Seizure 1996; 5: 235–8.
10. Nashef L, Walker F, Allen P et al. Apnea and bradycardia during epileptic seizures: relation to sudden death in epilepsy. J Neurol Neurosurg Psychiatry 1996; 60: 297–300.
11. Linzer M, Grubb BP, Ho S et al. Cardiovascular causes of loss of consciousness in patients with presumed epilepsy: a cause of the increased sudden death rate in people with epilepsy? Am J Med 1994; 96: 146–54.
12. Byard RW, Cutz E. Sudden and unexpected death in infancy and childhood due to pulmonary thromboembolism: an autopsy study. Arch Pathol Lab Med 1990; 114: 142–4.
13. Shemie S, Jay V, Rutka J, Armstrong D. Acute obstructive hydrocephalus and sudden death in children. Ann Emerg Med 1997; 29: 524–8.
14. SoRelle R. Jump in sudden deaths reported in younger people during the last decade. Circulation 2001; 103: E9019–21.
15. Myerburg RJ, Mitrami R, Interion A et al. Identification of risk of cardiac arrest and sudden death in athletes. In: Wang PG, ed. Sudden Cardiac Death in Athletes. Armonk, NY: Futura, 1998: 25–56.
16. Frommelt PC, Berger S, Pelech AN, Bergstrom S, Williamson JG. Prospective identification of anomalous origin of left coronary artery from the right sinus of Valsalva using transthoracic echocardiography: importance of color Doppler flow mapping. Pediatr Cardiol 2001; 22: 327–32.

17. Roberts WC, Shirani J. The four subtypes of anomalous origin of the left main coronary artery from the right aortic sinus (or from right coronary artery). Am J Cardiol 1992; 70: 119–21.
18. Barth CW, Roberts WC. Left main coronary artery originating from right sinus of Valsalva and coursing between the aorta and pulmonary trunk. J Am Coll Cardiol 1986; 7: 366–73.
19. Roberts WC, Siegel RJ, Zipes DP. Origin of the right coronary artery from left sinus of Valsalva and its functional consequences: analysis of ten necropsy patients. Am J Cardiol 1982; 49: 863–8.
20. McManus BM, Gries LA, Ness MJ. Anomalous origin of the right coronary artery from left sinus of Valsalva. Pediatr Pathol 1990; 10: 987–91.
21. Yamanaka O, Hobbs RE. Coronary artery anomalies in 126 595 patients undergoing coronary arteriography. Cathet Cardiovasc Diagn 1990; 21: 28–40.
22. Taylor AJ, Rogan KM, Virmani R. Sudden cardiac death associated with isolated congenital coronary artery anomalies. J Am Coll Cardiol 1992; 20: 640–7.
23. Frommelt PC, Frommelt MA, Tweddel JS, Jaquiss RD. Prospective echocardiographic diagnosis and surgical repair of anomalous origin of a coronary artery from the opposite sinus with an interarterial course. J Am Coll Cardiol 2003; 42: 148–54.
24. Lipsett J, Byard RW, Carpenter BF, Jimenez CL, Bourne AJ. Anomalous coronary arteries arising from the aorta associated with sudden death in infancy and early childhood. An autopsy series. Arch Pathol Lab Med 1991; 115: 770–3.
25. Liberthson RR, Gang DL, Custer J. Sudden death in an infant with aberrant origin of the right coronary artery from the left sinus of Valsalva of the aorta: case report and review of the literature. Pediatr Cardiol 1983; 4: 45–8.
26. Frommelt PC, Frommelt MA. Congenital coronary artery anomalies. Pediatr Clin North Am 2004; 51: 1273–88.
27. Shirani J, Roberts WC. Solitary coronary ostium in the aorta in the absence of other major congenital cardiovascular anomaly. J Am Coll Cardiol 1993; 21: 137–43.
28. Roberts WC. Major anomalies of coronary arterial origin seen in childhood. Am Heart J 1986; 111: 941–63.
29. Gay F, Vouhe P, Lecompte Y et al. Atresie de l'ostium coronaire gauche: réparation chez un nourison de deux mois. Arch Mal Coeur Vaiss 1989; 82: 807–10.
30. Bird LM, Billman G, Lacro R et al. Sudden death in Williams syndrome. Report of ten cases. J Pediatr 1986; 129: 926–31.
31. van Pelt NC, Wilson NJ, Lear G. Severe coronary artery disease in the absence of supravalvular stenosis in a patient with Williams syndrome. Pediatr Cardiol 2005; 26: 665–7.
32. Furuyama H, Odagawa Y, Katoh C et al. Altered myocardial flow reserve and endothelial function late after Kawasaki disease. J Pediatr 2003; 142: 149–54.
33. Maron BJ. Hypertrophic cardiomyopathy: a systematic review. JAMA 2002; 287: 1308–20.
34. Yertman AT, Hamilton RM, Benson LN, McRidle BW. Long term outcome and prognostic determinant in children with hypertrophic cardiomyopathy. J Am Coll Cardiol 1998; 32: 1943–50.
35. Arola A, Jokinen E, Ruuskanen O et al. Epidemiology of idiopathic cardiomyopathy in children and adolescents. A nationwide study in Finland. Am J Epidemiol 1997; 146: 385–93.
36. Towbin JA. Molecular genetic basis of sudden cardiac death. Pediatr Clin North Am 2004; 51: 1229–55.
37. Friedmann RA, Moak JP, Garson A. Clinical course of idiopathic dilated cardiomyopathy in children. J Am Coll Cardiol 1991; 18: 152–6.
38. Muller G, Ulmer HE, Hagel KJ, Wolf D. Cardiac dysrhythmias in children with idiopathic dilated or hypertrophic cardiomyopathy. Pediatr Cardiol 1995; 16: 56–60.
39. Rivenes SN, Kearney DL, O'Brian Smith E, Towbin JA, Denfield SW. Sudden death and cardiovascular collapse in children with restrictive cardiomyopathy. Circulation 2000; 102: 876–82.

40. Thiene G, Nava A, Corrado D, Rossi N, Pennelli N. Right ventricular cardiomyopathy and sudden death in young people. N Engl J Med 1988; 318: 129–33.
41. Lambert EC, Menon VR, Wagner HR, Vlad P. Sudden unexpected death from cardiovascular disease in children. A cooperative international study. Am J Cardiol 1974; 34: 89–96.
42. Garson A Jr, McNamara DG. Sudden death in a pediatric cardiologic population; 1958 to 1983: relation to prior arrhythmias. J Am Coll Cardiol 1985; 5: 134B–7B.
43. Silka MJ, Hardy GB, Menashe VD, Morris CD. A population-based prospective evaluation of risk of sudden cardiac death after operation for common congenital heart defects. J Am Coll Cardiol 1998; 32: 245–51.
44. Bastianon V, Del Bolgia F, Boscioni M et al. Altered cardiac repolarization during exercise in congenital aortic stenosis. Pediatr Cardiol 1993; 14: 23–7.
45. Wolfe RR, Driscoll DJ, Gersony WM et al. Arrhythmias in patients with valvar aortic stenosis, valvar pulmonary stenosis, and ventricular septal defects. Circulation 1993; 87: 89–101.
46. Murphy JG, Gersh BJ, Mair DD et al. Long-term outcome in patients undergoing surgical repair of tetralogy of Fallot. N Engl J Med 1993; 18: 93–9.
47. Puley G, Siu S, Connelly M et al. Arrhythmias and survival in patients >18 years of age after the Mustard procedure for complete transposition of great arteries. Am J Cardiol 1999; 83: 1080–4.
48. Sarkar D, Bull C, Yates R et al. Comparison of long-term outcomes of atrial repair of simple transposition with implication for a late arterial switch strategy. Circulation 1999; 100: II-176–II-81.
49. Losay J, Touchot A, Serraf A et al. Late outcome after arterial switch operation for transposition of great arteries. Circulation 2001; 104: I-121–I-6.
50. Celermajer DS, Cullen S, Sullivan ID et al. Outcome in neonates with Ebstein's anomaly. J Am Coll Cardiol 1992; 19: 1041–6.
51. Davos CH, Francis DP, Leenarts MFE et al. Global impairment of cardiac autonomic nervous activity late after the Fontan operation. Circulation 2003; 108: II-180–II-5.
52. Balaji S, Johnson TB, Sade RM, Case CL, Gillette PC. Management of atrial flutter after the Fontan procedure. J Am Coll Cardiol 1994; 23: 1209–15.
53. Vincent GM, Timothy KW, Leppert M, Keating M. The spectrum of symptom and QT interval in carriers of the genes for the long QT syndrome. New Engl J Med 1992; 327: 846–52.
54. Vincent GM. The molecular genetic of the long QT syndrome: gene causing fainting and sudden death. Annu Rev Med 1998; 49: 263–74.
55. Ackerman MJ. The long QT syndrome: ion channel diseases of the heart. Mayo Clin Proc 1998; 73: 250–69.
56. Andelfinger G, Tapper AR, Welch RC et al. KCNJ2 mutation results in Andersen syndrome with sex-specific cardiac and skeletal muscle phenotypes. Am J Hum Genet 2002; 71: 663–8.
57. Brugada P, Brugada J. Right bundle branch block, persistent ST segment elevation and sudden cardiac death: a distinct clinical and electrocardiographic syndrome. A multicenter report. J Am Coll Cardiol 1992; 20; 1391–6.
58. Priori SG, Napolitano C, Gasparini M et al. Clinical and genetic heterogeneity of right bundle branch block and ST-segment elevation syndrome: a prospective evaluation of 52 families. Circulation 2000; 102: 2509–15.
59. Leenhardt A, Lucet V, Denjoy I et al. Catecholaminergic polymorphic ventricular tachycardia in children: a seven year follow-up of 21 patients. Circulation 1995; 91: 1512–9.
60. Lahat H, Pras E, Eldar M. RYR2 and CASQ2 mutations in patients suffering from catecholaminergic polymorphic ventricular tachycardia. Circulation 2003; 107: e29.
61. Torner Montoya P, Brugada P, Smeets J et al. Ventricular fibrillation in the Wolff–Parkinson–White syndrome. Eur Heart J 1991; 12: 144–50.
62. Zangwill SD, Strasburger JF. Commotio cordis. Pediatr Clin North Am 2004; 51: 1347–54.
63. Link MS, Wang PJ, Pandian NG et al. Experimental model of sudden death due to low-energy chest wall impact (commotio cordis). N Engl J Med 1998; 338: 1805–11.

64. Isner JM, Estes M, Thompson PD et al. Acute cardiac events temporally related to cocaine abuse. N Engl J Med 1986; 315: 1438–43.
65. Isner JM, Roberts WC, Heymsfield SB, Yager J. Anorexia nervosa and sudden death. Ann Intern Med 1985; 102: 49–52.
66. Cina SJ, Smiallek JE, Burke AP, Virmanier R, Hutchins GM. Primary cardiac tumors causing sudden death. Review of the literature. Am J Forensic Med Pathol 1996; 17: 271–81.

# 11

# Inherited arrhythmia: present and future perspectives for genetic therapy

Silvia G Priori and Carlo Napolitano

## INTRODUCTION

Since the inception of the molecular cardiology era, cloning and molecular analysis of ion channels have shown that several clinical disorders primarily presenting with arrhythmia and sudden death (e.g., long-QT syndrome (LQTS), catecholaminergic polymorphic ventricular tachycardia (CPVT), familial atrial fibrillation) are due to genetically determined alterations of ionic fluxes (www.fsm.it/cardmoc). Hence, inherited arrhythmogenic diseases have become a sort of natural model that scientists exploit to investigate the molecular bases of cardiac excitability.

The logical next step is to develop novel approaches to correct the molecular substrates, that is, to find novel therapies for arrhythmia and sudden death. Two major strategies are being followed: 'gene-specific therapy' and 'gene therapy'. Gene-specific therapy is accomplished by selecting and testing drugs that have the potential to counteract the affected pathway causing the clinical phenotype. On the other hand, 'gene therapy' aims at directly replacing the defective gene with a healthy copy. *In vitro* gene transfer techniques are being developed, and many 'proof of concept studies' have shown that this approach is feasible, although the clinical applicability of gene therapy is still in its infancy.

Here we will summarize the clinical features and the pathogenesis of those arrhythmogenic diseases that have so far been considered amenable to gene-specific therapy. We will also discuss the current strategies that are being followed to develop gene therapy for cardiac arrhythmia.

## THE LONG-QT SYNDROME (LQTS)

The main features of LQTS are the abnormally prolonged cardiac repolarization (QT interval), abnormal T-wave morphology, and life-threatening cardiac arrhythmia. Cardiac events are often precipitated by physical or emotional stress. Therefore, antiadrenergic treatment with beta-blockers has been proposed and shown to be effective thereafter. Today, this approach still represents the cornerstone of therapy for LQTS. The unresponsive patients are candidates for implantable cardioverter defibrillator (ICD) and/or cardiac sympathetic denervation (LCSD). Recently, it has become evident that molecular genetics has an important role in this scenario thanks to genotype–phenotype correlation studies that have provided informative hints for locus-specific risk stratification and therapy.

### Genetic bases of LQTS

As of today, eight LQTS-related genes have been identified: five genes cause 'isolated' LQTS, and three cause QT interval prolongation and arrhythmia in the setting of a multiorgan disease (Andersen syndrome and Timothy syndrome) or with peculiar electrocardiographic manifestation (LQT4 – see below). The five genes causing the prototypical isolated LQTS are as follows: *KCNQ1* (LQT1), *KCNH2* (LQT2), *SCN5A* (LQT3),[1–3] *KCNE1* (LQT5)[4] and *KCNE2* (LQT6).[5] The two LQTS variants with extracardiac involvement, Andersen syndrome (LQT7) and Timothy syndrome (LQT8), have been linked to *KCNJ2*[6] and *CACNA1c*[7] mutations, respectively.

All the LQT1-3 and LQT5-8 genes encode for cardiac ion channel subunits. The exception is LQT4 due to mutations in the *ANK2* gene: an intracellular protein called ankyrin B that is involved in ion channel anchoring and localization to the plasmalemma.[8]

Molecular epidemiology data[9] show that nearly 70% of clinically affected subjects carry mutation in one known LQTS gene and approximately 95% of genetically affected patients carry a mutation in one of the three most frequent genes (*KCNQ1*, *KCNH2* and *SCN5A*). As a consequence, robust genotype-phenotype and physiopathologic data, useful for clinical management and locus-specific therapy, are available only for these variants.

### Functional consequences of genetic defects

Knowing the molecular pathophysiology of a disease is the first step to the development of specific therapy. In LQTS, ventricular repolarization is abnormal due to the action potential prolongation occurring at the cellular level. This effect may be obtained through either a reduction of the outward repolarizing or an excess of inward depolarizing currents. Both mechanisms turned out to occur in LQTS.

*KCNQ1* (LQT1) and *KCNE1* (LQT5) encode for the alpha- and the beta-subunits of the $I_{Ks}$ potassium channel[10] (Table 11.1), the slow component of the delayed rectifier current ($I_K$), the major repolarizing current during phase 3 of the cardiac action potential. *KCNQ1*-related LQTS is the most common variant and over 150 different mutations have been reported (http://www.fsm.it/cardmoc). This alpha-subunit is a transmembrane protein with six membrane-spanning segments. In order to make a functional channel, alpha-subunits form homotetramers, and they coassemble with beta-subunits *KCNE1*, a small protein with a single transmembrane segment.

A similar topology and assembling pattern is reported for *KCNH2* (LQT2) and *KCNE2* (LQT6) genes, encoding for the alpha- and the beta-subunits of the $I_{Kr}$ potassium channel, the rapid component of the cardiac delayed rectifier.[5,11] LQT2 is the second most common variant of LQTS, accounting for 35–40% of patients. Conversely, mutations of the *KCNE2* gene cause LQT6,[5] which is a very uncommon variant of the disease (<1% of genotyped patients).

*SCN5A* (LQT3) mutations are identified in approximately 10% of genotyped LQTS patients.[9,12] This gene encodes for the alpha-subunit of the cardiac sodium channel, a transmembrane protein composed of four homologous domains (DI–DIV), each containing six transmembrane segments (S1–S6). This alpha-subunit alone is able to conduct a current closely resembling the $I_{Na}$, although two auxiliary beta-subunits may modulate the ionic flux.[13]

**Table 11.1** Classification mechanisms and gene-specific therapies for inherited arrhythmogenic diseases

| Phenotype | Function | Variant | Gene | Protein | Functional alteration | Proposed gene-specific treatment |
|---|---|---|---|---|---|---|
| LQTS | $I_{Ks}$ potassium current | LQT1 | *KCNQ1* | $I_{Ks}$ potassium channel alpha-subunit (KvLQT1) | Loss of function | None |
| | | LQT5 | *KCNE1* | $I_{Ks}$ potassium channel beta-subunit (MinK) | Loss of function | |
| | $I_{Kr}$ potassium current | LQT2 | *KCNH* | $I_{Kr}$ potassium channel alpha-subunit (HERG) | Loss of function | • Increase $I_{Kr}$ ≥1.5 mEq/l above baseline: potassium supplements |
| | | LQT6 | *KCNE2* | $I_{Kr}$ potassium channel beta-subunit (MiRP) | Loss of function | • Rescue of trafficking: fexofenadine, thapsigargin |
| | $I_{Na}$ sodium current | LQT3 | *SCN5A* | Cardiac sodium channel alpha-subunit (Nav 1.5) | Gain of function | • Block of $I_{Na}$: mexiletine |
| Brugada syndrome | $I_{Na}$ sodium current | BrS1 | *SCN5A* | Cardiac sodium channel alpha-subunit (Nav 1.5) | Loss of function | • Block of $I_{To}$: quinidine, tedisamil, cilostazol<br>• Rescue of trafficking-defective mutants: mexiletine |
| CPVT | | CPVT1 | *RyR2* | Cardiac ryanodine receptor (RyR2) | Gain of function | • Recovery of FKBP12.6 binding: JTV519 |
| | | CPVT2 | *CASQ2* | Cardiac calsequestrin | Loss of function | — |

*KCNJ2*, the gene responsible for Andersen syndrome (LQT7), encodes for Kir2.1, a two-transmembrane segments protein that tetramerizes to form functional channels. *KCNJ2* controls the $I_{K1}$ current (also referred to as inward rectifier), an important player during the late repolarization phase and for the resting membrane potential control.[14]

The potassium channel-dependent LQTS is due to loss of function mutations (Table 11.1).[15] Expression of mutant proteins in heterologous cellular systems has consistently shown that the final effect of mutation is an abnormal slowing of cardiac repolarization. However, there are multiple biophysical mechanisms leading to such repolarization impairment. The integration of mutant proteins may be deleterious and even alter the function of the protein produced by the wild-type allele: a dominant negative effect, resulting in >50% reduction of current. In some instances, the defective (mutant) proteins are retained in the Golgi apparatus (trafficking defect). In such instances, the functional defect is mainly due to the 'lack' of proteins (those produced by the mutant allele) that determines a 50% current reduction (haploinsufficiency).[15] Rescue of trafficking is one of the possible gene-specific strategies for loss of function potassium channel mutations (see below).

*SCN5A* (LQT3) and *CACNA1c* (Timothy syndrome, LQT8) mutations are caused by 'gain-of-function' mutation, causing an excess of depolarizing force leading to action potential prolongation with an opposite mechanism as compared with potassium-dependent LQTS. Several electrophysiologic consequences of LQT3 mutants have been identified: late sustained current, slower inactivation, faster recovery from inactivation, and altered interaction with beta 1-subunit.[15] The calcium channel mutation G408R found in Timothy syndrome causes an almost complete loss of voltage dependence of the L-type calcium current, translating into a reduced current inactivation at all potential range during the cardiac cycle.

## Genotype–phenotype correlation and risk stratification

Genotype-specific T-wave patterns and triggers for cardiac events have been reported by several authors[16–18] (Figure 11.1). Albeit not a surrogate to genetic testing, these features may be important to define the genotyping strategy and for counselling patients.

Even more relevant is the possibility of combining the genotype with 'traditional' clinical variables (ECG, personal and familial history of cardiac events and gender) to reach clinically applicable risk-stratification schemes. Priori et al showed that the combination of QTc duration, genotype and gender modulates the natural history of the disease.[19] These authors showed that, among LQT1 and LQT2, those with a QTc in the upper quartile (>500 ms) have a 5.3- and 8.4-fold risk increase, respectively, as compared with those in the first quartile. Gender has no influence among LQT1 patients, whereas a higher risk is demonstrated for LQT2 if patients are female and for LQT3 if male.

In smaller patients' groups, it has been suggested that risk stratification may be further refined, including the position of the mutation in the predicted membrane topology of the involved protein. Pore region mutation of *KCNH2* may bear an increased risk of events,[20] while the carboxy-terminus *KCNQ1* mutations could be associated with mild phenotype and low penetrance.[21,22] Although intriguing, these latter results are still under discussion and they require further investigation before reaching full clinical applicability.

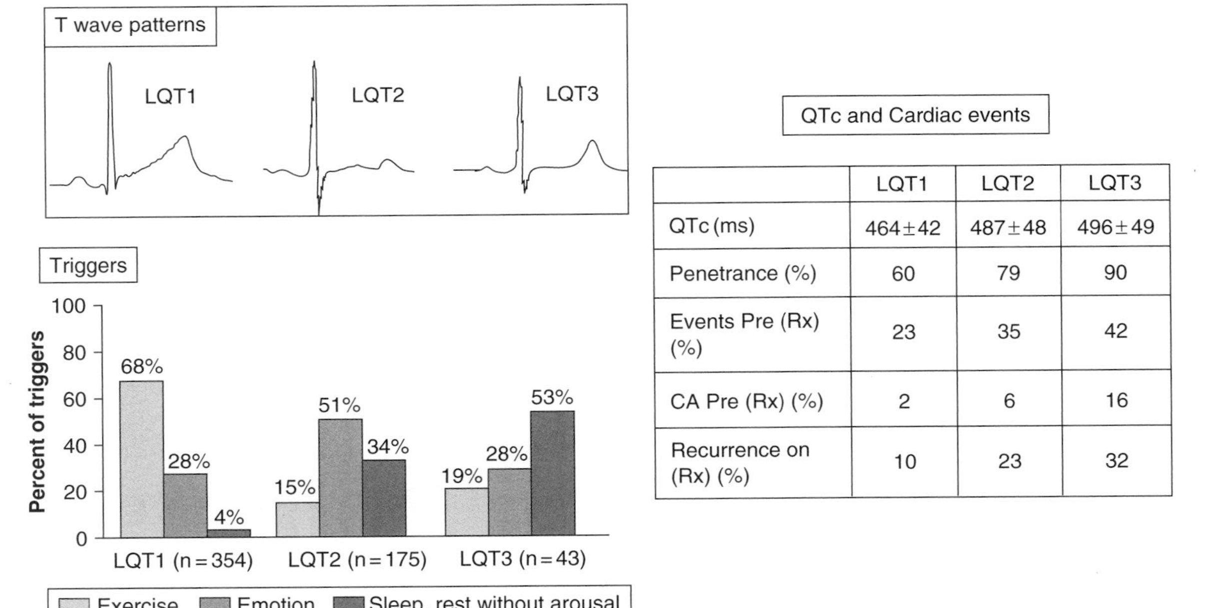


| | LQT1 | LQT2 | LQT3 |
|---|---|---|---|
| QTc (ms) | 464±42 | 487±48 | 496±49 |
| Penetrance (%) | 60 | 79 | 90 |
| Events Pre (Rx) (%) | 23 | 35 | 42 |
| CA Pre (Rx) (%) | 2 | 6 | 16 |
| Recurrence on (Rx) (%) | 10 | 23 | 32 |

**Figure 11.1** Genotype-specific phenotype in LQTS. The figure summarizes the most important genotype-phenotype correlation data in LQTS having an impact on clinical management. Specific ST–T-wave patterns (upper-left panel) consist of broad-based and smooth T wave, low amplitude and notched T wave, straight ST segment and small peaked T wave in LQT1, LQT2 and LQT3, respectively. Triggers for cardiac events (lower-left panel) clearly distinguish LQT1 patients having the majority of events during physical activity from LQT3 patients, who usually have syncope and cardiac arrest during rest or sleep (modified from Schwartz et al[17]). QTc and natural history also show genotype-specific behavior (right panel): LQT2 and LQT3 patients have longer QTc and higher incidence of events and significantly higher recurrence rate of events on therapy (Rx) than LQT1 patients (data from Priori et al[19] and Priori et al[25]).

## Therapy

*Genotype-specific targeting of standard therapies in LQTS*

The mainstay of LQTS therapy is represented by beta-blockers,[23] which are indicated in all patients with clinically overt phenotype, with or without history of syncope. ICD plus beta-blockade is indicated for secondary prevention, in patients with an aborted cardiac arrest and in those experiencing a recurrent cardiac event on therapy.[24]

In a recent study, we demonstrated that genotype also significantly modulates the effectiveness of therapy.[25] Indeed, beta-blockers are significantly more effective among LQT1 than LQT2 (relative risk vs LQT1 2.81; 95% CI: 1.50–5.27) and LQT3 (relative risk vs LQT1 4.00; 95% CI: 2.45–8.03) patients. In this study, additional independent predictors of cardiac events on therapy were the presence of a first cardiac event before therapy in early childhood (≤7 years) and a QTc interval of >500 ms. Thus, LQT2 and LQT3 patients with a QTc interval longer than 500 ms are at high risk of events despite active beta-blockade and might be candidates for more aggressive treatment such as primary prevention with ICD.

Another clinically relevant issue that progressively emerged after the discovery of LQTS genes is that of silent mutation carriers. These individuals, representing approximately 30% of all genotyped LQTS patients, despite a normal QT interval, still present an approximately 10% risk of cardiac events before age 40.[19] Thus, beta-blocking therapy in these individuals may be considered.

*Gene-specific therapy*

*Gene-specific targeting of loss-of-function potassium channel mutations* While, at present, no attempts have been made specifically to counteract the detrimental effects of mutations in *KCNQ1* (LQT1) and *KCNJ2*, approaches to correct the consequence of *KNCH2* (LQT2) mutants have been extensively explored. This line of research is clinically justified by the fact that these latter patients, unlike those with LQT1, are quite refractory to treatment with beta-blockers.[25]

*Potassium control* Conductance of *KCNH2* channels is directly related to extracellular $[K^+]$.[11] Based on this evidence, Compton et al[26] hypothesized that increasing extracellular $[K^+]$ by oral potassium supplements could enhance the amount of current and at least partially compensate for the loss of current induced by *KCNH2* mutations. In a pilot clinical study, these authors showed that a ≥1.5 mEq/l increase of plasma $[K^+]$ above baseline yields a QT interval shortening close to the normal level.[26] A prospective clinical trial is now underway to assess whether, besides shortening repolarization, potassium supplements can also prevent cardiac arrhythmia in carriers of *KCNH2* mutations.

*Rescue of defective trafficking* Defective intracellular trafficking of *KCNQ1* and *KCNH2* mutants is an important pathophysiologic mechanism in LQT2.[15]

In 1999, Zhou et al[27] demonstrated that culturing cells at lower temperature (27°C instead of 37°C) or in the presence of compounds such as E4031, astemizole, or cisapride, restores the trafficking into the plasma membrane of *KCNH2* mutants. Unfortunately, these compounds are also blockers of the same channel, and the two effects (rescue of trafficking and channel blockade) occur at similar concentrations. As a consequence, the benefit provided by the rescue of protein trafficking is diminished by the channel blockade.[27] Subsequently, other drugs have been tested in the attempt to separate the effect on trafficking from that of channel blockade, and two agents were found to be particularly promising: fexofenadine, a metabolite of terfenadine,[28] and thapsigargin, an inhibitor of the SERCA pump.[29] Both agents showed a significant restoration of trafficking without current blocking effect. Taken together, these studies suggest that it is possible to dissociate the two effects (channel blocking activity and trafficking correction), bringing this strategy closer to clinical applicability (Table 11.1).

*Gene-specific targeting of gain-of-function SCN5A mutations* Sodium channel blockade represents a rational approach for a gene-specific therapy in LQT3 (Table 11.1), since mutations induce an excess of sodium entering into the cells during phase 0 (depolarization) of cardiac action potential. Preliminary experimental and clinical evidence shows that mexiletine up to 10 mg/kg per day effectively shortens the action potential and the QT interval.[30,31] Furthermore, short-term efficacy of mexiletine to prevent lethal events has been reported,[32,33] although there are no prospective data demonstrating that mexiletine improves long-term survival in LQT3 patients.

Interestingly, experimental observations have suggested that the efficacy of $I_{Na}$ blockade may be mutation-specific,[34] and the same mutation may not respond equally to different sodium channel blockers. For instance, the effects of D1790G are selectively counteracted by flecainide, but not by lidocaine, during repetitive stimulation (use-dependent block).[35]

Clinical experience suggests that the sodium channel blocker, flecainide, should be used with caution in LQT3 patients, since it may induce ST-segment elevation, resembling a Brugada syndrome ECG, in approximately 50% of cases when administered to unselected LQT3 patients.[36] The use of flecainide in LQT3 should be limited to patients for whom the lack of ST segment elevation is clearly demonstrated.

Thus, sodium channel blockade is a rational and promising treatment of LQT3 patients. The experimental findings suggest that there could be a mutation-specific effect and that not all $I_{Na}$ blockers are equally effective, indicating that there are still knowledge gaps to fill.[34,35] Nonetheless, the clinical data suggest that mexiletine may be used as an adjunctive treatment to beta-blockade or to the ICD to prevent cardiac events in high-risk LQT3 patients.

## BRUGADA SYNDROME (BrS)

Brugada syndrome (BrS) is clinically characterized by peculiar ECG alterations (ST-segment elevation in leads V1–V3 and complete or incomplete right-bundle branch block) and risk of sudden cardiac death (SCD) due to the onset of fast polymorphic ventricular tackycardia (VT) and ventricular fibrillation.[37] BrS is often inherited as autosomal dominant trait, even if a high prevalence of sporadic cases is encountered in the clinical practice.

Diagnosis of BrS may be complicated by the transitory nature of the ECG abnormalities.[38,39] Provocative testing with intravenous administration of sodium channel blockers (flecainide 2 mg/kg or ajamaline 1 mg/kg) may help unmask the ECG abnormalities in suspected cases, but its sensitivity is yet undefined.[40] The ST-segment morphology is also a matter of debate, and criteria have been modified over time. In the earlier reports, BrS diagnosis was considered in the presence of both a 'coved' and a 'saddleback' ECG pattern.[41] Subsequently,[42] only coved ECG (either spontaneous or pharmacologically induced) has been reported as diagnostic for the disease. In 2005, even more restrictive criteria were introduced in a consensus document,[43] in which the presence of a coved ECG was not considered sufficient for diagnosis in the absence of additional criteria such as programmed electrical stimulation (PES) inducibility and ventricular arrhythmia (syncope or cardiac arrest). It is fair to recall that this definition is questioned by the results of genotype-phenotype analyses showing that carriers of loss-of-function mutation may have a 'saddleback' ECG and may remain asymptomatic, or ventricular arrhythmias may not be induced at PES.[40]

### Genetic bases

After the initial report in 1998,[44] tens of different BrS mutations have been reported (http://www.fsm.it/cardmoc). Unfortunately, *SCN5A* underlies no more than 20–25% of clinical cases.[45] Another BrS locus was mapped in a 5 cM region (i.e. a region of chromosome encompassing 5 million nucleotides) on chromosome 3p22–25 in a large family with autosomal dominant inheritance, but so far the gene responsible for BrS at this locus remains unknown. The limited knowledge on the genetic bases of BrS currently hampers clinically useful genotype–phenotype correlation.

Therefore, the clinical decision-making process and the risk stratification must be done on a clinical basis. Nonetheless, genetic testing, when successful, allows us to confirm the diagnosis in borderline cases, to identify silent carriers and to assess the reproductive risk.

### Functional consequences of genetic mutations

Functional expression studies showed a spectrum of biophysical abnormalities leading to a loss of function of the cardiac sodium channel,[15,46] such as: 1) failure of the channel to express (haploinsufficiency, with trafficking defect); 2) shift of voltage- and time-dependent channel activation, inactivation or reactivation; 3) entry of $I_{Na}$ into an intermediate, slowly recovering, state of inactivation; 4) acceleration of inactivation.

### Therapy

#### *Standard approach*

BrS presents with syncope and cardiac arrest typically in the third and fourth decades of life, and usually at rest or during sleep. At present, there is no effective pharmacologic treatment to prevent arrhythmia and the ICD is the only option for high-risk individuals. For this reason, the standard approach to therapy requires careful risk stratification to limit device implantation in those 20% of the BrS patients who will experience at least one life-threatening cardiac event in their lifetime.[47,48]

Of course, the development of a pharmacologic approach to counteract the electrophysiologic abnormalities induced by mutations also would mean a remarkable improvement of clinical management.

While the use of the ICD for secondary prevention of aborted cardiac arrest is clearly indicated, the correct strategy for identification of high-risk patients in whom the ICD is justified as primary prevention is still debated.

In 2002, we showed that the presence of a spontaneous ST-segment elevation in leads V1, V2, and/or V3, especially when associated with a history of syncope, was the most robust indicator of risk of cardiac events.[45] This concept was subsequently confirmed by other investigators.[47] On the other hand, the ICD indications for asymptomatic (i.e., no syncope in the clinical history) patients remain controversial. This group has a relatively low risk of cardiac events (10–15%).[45,49] Although PES has been proposed as a valuable risk-stratification tool, other authors have not confirmed this hypothesis.[45,49] Therefore, the issue of identifying robust marker for this subgroup of patients remains open.

### *Gene-specific therapy*

Quinidine, a nonspecific blocker of cardiac transient outward current ($I_{to}$), has been proposed as gene-specific therapy for BrS (Table 11.1). This proposal is based on the idea that the loss of sodium inward current tilts the balance between outward and inward currents, with an abnormal shift in the outward direction at the end of phase 1 of the action potential. Since transmural distribution of transient inward current is not uniform, this condition creates a dispersion of repolarization and arrhythmogenic substrate.[50] The block of repolarizing currents, and specifically $I_{to}$, which is active during the initial phases of action potential, could restore the equilibrium.[51] Based on this appealing theory, some authors have attempted a gene-specific approach to therapy in BrS.

The available clinical data show that quinidine prevents inducibility of arrhythmia at PES in up to 76% of BrS patients[52–54] and suggest a positive long-term effect in preventing the occurrence of spontaneous arrhythmia.[54] Unfortunately, the high incidence of gastrointestinal side effects may reduce patient compliance.[54] Tedisamil, a novel anti-ischemic and antiarrhythmic drug, still in the premarketing phase, has been proposed as an alternative to quinidine in BrS patients,[55] but clinical data are not yet available.

Cilostazol, an oral phosphodiesterase III inhibitor marketed as an antiplatelet agent, has been used in a single BrS patient, in whom it normalized the ST segment and prevented the occurrence of ventricular fibrillation.[56] Cilostazol increases $I_{Ca}$ by inhibiting phosphodiesterase activity in ventricular myocytes, and it decreases $I_{to}$ (Table 11.2).

Overall, these approaches to gene-specific therapy of BrS involve the block of $I_{to}$ current. The available data suggest a possible clinical efficacy only for quinidine. This treatment should be currently regarded as an adjunctive treatment to ICD in the attempt to reduce the number of device interventions for high-risk patients, and not as a first-line therapy.

### *Rescue of defective trafficking*

Trafficking-defective mutants have been also identified in *SCN5A* and associated with BrS.[57,58] Interestingly, mexiletine was able to restore $I_{Na}$ by rescuing the proper localization of the protein[57] (Table 11.1). However, mexiletine also blocks the sodium channel (see above under 'Gene-specific targetting of gain-of-function *SCN5A* mutations'), which, of course, is not desirable for BrS therapy. Whether the separation of channel blocking effect from trafficking restoration is possible has not been determined so far.

## CATECHOLAMINERGIC POLYMORPHIC VENTRICULAR TACHYCARDIA (CPVT)

CPVT is an arrhythmic disorder clinically characterized by VT syncope and sudden death occurring in familial as well as sporadic cases.[59] The three distinguishing features are 1) direct relationship between adrenergic activation (physical or emotional stress) and the onset of arrhythmia; 2) typical pattern of bidirectional VT, with an unremarkable resting ECG and 3) structurally normal heart.[59]

The onset of ventricular arrhythmia during exercise reproducible in terms of onset heart rate (120–130 beats/min) and morphology (the so-called bidirectional VT: a 180° QRS axis alternans on a beat-to-beat basis). In some instances, however, polymorphic VT without a 'stable' QRS vector alternans may be observed.[60,61]

CPVT usually appears with syncope triggered by exercise or acute emotion, although SCD may be the first manifestation in some families.[61] In the absence of appropriate therapy, more than 70% of patients experience syncope or aborted cardiac arrest before the age of 40 years.[62] Symptoms often appear during childhood with a mean age of first event of 8 years, and approximately 30% of families present with one or more premature sudden deaths that usually occur during childhood, although later events may also occur (after age 20).[61,63]

### Genetic bases

On the basis of previous linkage mapping data in 2001, we identified the cardiac ryanodine receptor gene *RyR2* as the gene involved in the pathogenesis of CPVT.[64] The ryanodine receptor is the most important $Ca^{2+}$-releasing channel in the cardiac sarcoplasmic reticulum (SR). It localizes across the membrane of the SR, and it releases $Ca^{2+}$ in response to the calcium entry through the L-type channels (Cav1.2). Experimental data suggest that CPVT mutations destabilize the protein with consequent $Ca^{2+}$ overload, thus facilitating the occurrence of delayed afterdepolarization (DAD).[65,66]

A rare autosomal recessive variant of CPVT has also been described and linked to the *CASQ2* gene on chromosome 1p11–p13. This gene encodes for calsequestrin, and it is involved in $Ca^{2+}$ homeostasis by serving the major $Ca^{2+}$-buffering protein into the SR cisternae.

The amount of clinical and genetic data available does not allow us to draw robust genotype–phenotype correlation and risk-stratification algorithms. CPVT patients are usually not inducible at programmed electrical stimulation, making it inadequate for management and risk stratification.[61,63] Preliminary evidence shows that patients with RyR2 mutation have events at a younger age than do patients with nongenotyped CPVT and that male sex is a risk factor for syncope in RyR2-CPVT (relative risk=4.2).[61] The clinical presentation of *CASQ2*-and *RyR2*-related CPVT is similar, although it has been suggested that CASQ2-CPVT most often presents with polymorphic instead of bidirectional VT.[67,68]

### Therapy

#### *Standard approach*

Antiadrenergic treatment with beta-blockers is the cornerstone of therapy for CPVT patients.[69] Chronic treatment with beta-blocking agents (e.g., Nadolol

1.5–2.5 mg/kg/per day) can prevent recurrence of syncope in the majority of patients.[61,63] The reproducible pattern of arrhythmia during the exercise stress test among CPVT patients allows dose titration and monitoring. Nonetheless, 40% of patients continue to show exercise-induced arrhythmia on maximal tolerated dose. In such instances, the use of an ICD appears indicated.[61]

*Gene-specific therapy*

One of the possible pathophysiologic mechanisms of *RyR2* mutations in CPVT is a decreased binding of calstabin 2 (a 'stabilizer' of the channel in the closed state, also known as FKBP12.6) to the RyR2 channel.[70] Interestingly, a similar mechanism has been proposed also for the pathogenesis of ventricular dysfunction and possibly SCD during heart failure.[71] In knockout calstabin-2 haploinsufficient (−/+) mice, the experimental agent JTV519, a 1,4-benzothiazepine derivative that favors the binding of calstabin 2 to RyR2,[71] has been shown to prevent the occurrence of ventricular arrhythmia.[72] Further *in vitro* experiments on a RyR2 mutant[70] showed that JTV519 restores the normal activity of the channel. These findings suggest that RyR2 stabilization in the closed state, by recovering calstabin 2 affinity, could represent a gene-specific therapy for CPVT (Table 11.1). However, other authors have suggested that the calstabin 2 pathway does not play a significant role in the pathogenesis of CPVT and have therefore questioned this gene-specific therapy approach. The availability of an animal model of CPVT[73] would allow us to assess whether JTV519 constitutes a potential therapy for CPVT.

## PERSPECTIVES FOR THE DEVELOPMENT OF GENE THERAPY OF CARDIAC ARRHYTHMIA

Gene-specific therapies (such as mexiletine for LQT3 patients and quinidine for BrS patients) are moving from the laboratory to initial clinical application. The availability of new models, such as expression of mutant proteins in cardiac myocytes and the use of transgenic animals, opens very promising perspectives for the further development of these novel therapies. However, gene therapy for cardiac arrhythmia and inherited arrhythmogenic disorders is in a much earlier stage of development.

Gene therapy seeks to replace the defective gene with a normal copy, thus providing a definitive cure for a specific disorder. This objective is still far from realization in clinical practice. Nonetheless, in recent years, myocardial gene transfer techniques have been progressively exploited and are approaching this final objective.

### Genetic modification of cardiac action potential (AP)

After physiologically important cardiac ion channels have been cloned and their relative contribution to action potential (AP) understood, several attempts have been made to modify the electrical milieu through over- or underexpression of transmembrane currents. The first successful attempts in using adenoviral vectors to modify AP by inducing the expression of potassium channels were reported in 1995 and 1996.[74,75] Several other studies followed, showing that gene therapy might be an attractive opportunity.[76] These studies also showed that in order to obtain a fine control of the cardiac excitability to the extent required for antiarrhythmic therapy, the molecular targeting of a single pathway is probably not sufficient given the complexity of the system.[76] Thus, a 'combined' approach is desirable. At least at the *in vitro* level, this has been achieved by some authors. For example, it has been shown that simultaneous overexpression of SERCA (sarcoplasmic reticulum ATPase) and Kv1.2 (potassium channel involved in the regulation of resting membrane potential) in cardiac myocytes shortens AP duration and increases the efficiency of calcium handling.[77] Other authors have attempted 'localized' gene therapy. Donahue et al[78,79] showed that *in vivo* overexpression of G protein in the atrioventricular node significantly reduces heart rate in an animal model of atrial fibrillation and reverses tachycardiomyopathy caused by the uncontrolled heart rate during chronic atrial fibrillation. Similarly, a positive effect on heart rate control during atrial fibrillation has been reported by Murata et al,[80] who developed a 'genetic' calcium antagonist by transduction of Gem, a ras-related G protein, which inhibits the trafficking of calcium channel alpha-subunits in the plasma membrane. Finally, *in vitro* and *in vivo* studies are now directed toward the development of 'biological pace-makers' that could compensate for a failing sinus node.[81]

Overall, these and other experiments have provided proof of the concept that modulation of AP duration by gene transfer is possible and that it may have beneficial effects. However, our capability to fine-tune cardiac AP by gene therapy is still in its infancy, and thus is not yet available in the clinical practice for the therapy of inherited arrhythmia.

### Current limitations in the field of gene therapy

Major problems in the field of gene therapy of cardiac arrhythmia (and gene therapy of cardiac disorders in general) are still to be solved: the low efficiency of gene transfer techniques, the lack of control of duration and level of transgene expression, and the potential immune responses generated by transfer vectors.

The inability to recruit all the cells in a targeted region is an important limitation for the gene therapy of cardiac arrhythmia. Indeed, this may result in heterogeneous modification of AP properties, thus resulting in a proarrhythmic rather than antiarrhythmic effect. Currently available gene-delivery techniques include direct DNA intramyocardial injection, delivery through the coronary arteries or epicardial administration. Overall these gene-delivery techniques are rather efficient for local delivery (up to 50% of transferred cells), when the goal is to modify the electrophysiologic substrate of a localized region (a few millimeters away from the point of injection), such as the atrioventricular node or pacemaker region.[76] However, the means to achieve homogeneous delivery throughout the myocardium is still not available.

The second relevant limitation concerns the time-limited expression of the transgene. At present, the effects of delivered genes are observed for no longer than 3–4 weeks, far too short a time to be considered for chronic disorders such as inherited arrhythmia, particularly when considering the invasive approach required for delivery. Many laboratories are actively working to improve vector efficiency and gene-delivery techniques, and it is expected that these problems will be solved in a few years.

## CONCLUSIONS

In the past decade, molecular biology has allowed us to elucidate the genetic background of several inherited diseases predisposing to cardiac arrhythmia and SCD. Functional characterization of mutant proteins has provided fascinating insights into the electrophysiologic derangements that account for the phenotypes. Now that genetics has entered clinical cardiology, playing a role in diagnosis and novel risk-stratification strategies, fundamental research has already set its next goal, and several groups are turning their attention to the development of locus-specific therapies. While direct correction of the defective gene through gene therapy is still in a preliminary phase, gene-specific therapies (e.g., mexiletine for LQT3 patients and quinidine for BrS patients) are moving from the laboratory to initial clinical applications. These rapid technological developments will certainly bring these approaches to the clinical arena.

## REFERENCES

1. Wang Q, Curran ME, Splawski I et al. Positional cloning of a novel potassium channel gene: KVLQT1 mutations cause cardiac arrhythmias. Nat Genet 1996; 12: 17–23.
2. Curran ME, Splawski I, Timothy KW et al. A molecular basis for cardiac arrhythmia: HERG mutations cause long QT syndrome. Cell 1995; 80: 795–803.
3. Wang Q, Shen J, Splawski I et al. SCN5A mutations associated with an inherited cardiac arrhythmia, long QT syndrome. Cell 1995; 80: 805–11.
4. Splawski I, Tristani-Firouzi M, Lehmann MH, Sanguinetti MC, Keating MT. Mutations in the hminK gene cause long QT syndrome and suppress IKs function. Nat Genet 1997; 17: 338–40.
5. Abbott GW, Sesti F, Splawski I et al. MiRP1 forms IKr potassium channels with HERG and is associated with cardiac arrhythmia. Cell 1999; 97: 175–87.
6. Plaster NM, Tawil R, Tristani-Firouzi M et al. Mutations in Kir2.1 cause the developmental and episodic electrical phenotypes of Andersen's syndrome. Cell 2001; 105: 511–9.
7. Splawski I, Timothy KW, Sharpe LM et al. Ca(V)1.2 calcium channel dysfunction causes a multisystem disorder including arrhythmia and autism. Cell 2004; 119: 19–31.
8. Mohler PJ, Schott JJ, Gramolini AO et al. Ankyrin-B mutation causes type 4 long-QT cardiac arrhythmia and sudden cardiac death. Nature 2003; 421: 634–9.
9. Napolitano C, Priori SG, Schwartz PJ et al. Genetic testing in the long QT syndrome: development and validation of an efficient approach to genotyping in the clinical practice. JAMA 2005; 294: 2975–80.
10. Barhanin J, Lesage F, Guillemare E et al. K(V)LQT1 and lsK (minK) proteins associate to form the I(Ks) cardiac potassium current. Nature 1996; 384: 78–80.
11. Sanguinetti MC, Jurkiewicz NK. Delayed rectifier outward $K^+$ current is composed of two currents in guinea pig atrial cells. Am J Physiol 1991; 260: H393–H9.
12. Splawski I, Shen J, Timothy KW et al. Spectrum of mutations in long-QT syndrome genes: KVLQT1, HERG, SCN5A, KCNE1, and KCNE2. Circulation 2000; 102: 1178–85.
13. Kupershmidt S, Yang T, Roden DM. Modulation of cardiac $Na^+$ current phenotype by beta1-subunit expression. Circ Res 1998; 83: 441–7.
14. Miake J, Marban E, Nuss HB. Functional role of inward rectifier current in heart probed by Kir2.1 overexpression and dominant-negative suppression. J Clin Invest 2003; 111: 1529–36.
15. Priori SG, Rivolta I, Napolitano C. Genetics of long QT, Brugada and other channellopathies. In: Zipes DP, Jalife J, eds. Cardiac Electrophysiology. 4th edn. Philadelphia: Elsevier, 2003: 462–70.
16. Moss AJ, Zareba W, Benhorin J et al. ECG T-wave patterns in genetically distinct forms of the hereditary long QT syndrome. Circulation 1995; 92: 2929–34.
17. Schwartz PJ, Priori SG, Spazzolini C et al. Genotype-phenotype correlation in the long-QT syndrome: gene-specific triggers for life-threatening arrhythmias. Circulation 2001; 103: 89–95.
18. Ali RH, Zareba W, Moss AJ et al. Clinical and genetic variables associated with acute arousal and nonarousal-related cardiac events among subjects with long QT syndrome. Am J Cardiol 2000; 85: 457–61.

19. Priori SG, Schwartz PJ, Napolitano C et al. Risk stratification in the long-QT syndrome. N Engl J Med 2003; 348: 1866–74.
20. Moss AJ, Zareba W, Kaufman ES et al. Increased risk of arrhythmic events in long-QT syndrome with mutations in the pore region of the human ether-a-go-go-related gene potassium channel. Circulation 2002; 105: 794–9.
21. Donger C, Denjoy I, Berthet M et al. KVLQT1 C-terminal missense mutation causes a forme fruste long-QT syndrome. Circulation 1997; 96: 2778–81.
22. Zareba W, Moss AJ, Sheu G et al. Location of mutation in the KCNQ1 and phenotypic presentation of long QT syndrome. J Cardiovasc Electrophysiol 2003; 14: 1149–53.
23. Moss AJ, Schwartz PJ, Crampton RS et al. The long QT syndrome. Prospective longitudinal study of 328 families. Circulation 1991; 84: 1136–44.
24. Moss AJ, Zareba W, Hall WJ et al. Effectiveness and limitations of beta-blocker therapy in congenital long-QT syndrome. Circulation 2000; 101: 616–23.
25. Priori SG, Napolitano C, Schwartz PJ et al. Association of long QT syndrome loci and cardiac events among patients treated with beta-blockers. JAMA 2004; 292: 1341–4.
26. Compton SJ, Lux RL, Ramsey MR et al. Genetically defined therapy of inherited long-QT syndrome. Correction of abnormal repolarization by potassium. Circulation 1996; 94: 1018–22.
27. Zhou Z, Gong Q, January CT. Correction of defective protein trafficking of a mutant HERG potassium channel in human long QT syndrome. Pharmacological and temperature effects. J Biol Chem 1999; 274: 31123–6.
28. Rajamani S, Anderson CL, Anson BD, January CT. Pharmacological rescue of human K(+) channel long-QT2 mutations: human ether-a-go-go-related gene rescue without block. Circulation 2002; 105: 2830–5.
29. Delisle BP, Anderson CL, Balijepalli RC et al. Thapsigargin selectively rescues the trafficking defective LQT2 channels G601S and F805C. J Biol Chem 2003; 278: 35749–54.
30. Priori SG, Napolitano C, Cantu F, Brown AM, Schwartz PJ. Differential response to $Na^+$ channel blockade, beta-adrenergic stimulation, and rapid pacing in a cellular model mimicking the SCN5A and HERG defects present in the long-QT syndrome. Circ Res 1996; 78: 1009–15.
31. Schwartz PJ, Priori SG, Locati EH et al. Long QT syndrome patients with mutations of the SCN5A and HERG genes have differential responses to $Na^+$ channel blockade and to increases in heart rate. Implications for gene-specific therapy. Circulation 1995; 92: 3381–6.
32. Schwartz PJ, Priori SG, Dumaine R et al. A molecular link between the sudden infant death syndrome and the long-QT syndrome. N Engl J Med 2000; 343: 262–7.
33. Kehl HG, Haverkamp W, Rellensmann G et al. Images in cardiovascular medicine. Life-threatening neonatal arrhythmia: successful treatment and confirmation of clinically suspected extreme long QT-syndrome-3. Circulation 2004; 109: e205–e6.
34. Rivolta I, Giarda E, Nastoli J et al. In vitro characterization of the electrophysiological effects of mexiletine on SCN5A mutants predicts clinical response in LQT3 patients. Circulation 110[17], III-230. 26-10-2004. Ref Type: Abstract.
35. Abriel H, Wehrens XH, Benhorin J, Kerem B, Kass RS. Molecular pharmacology of the sodium channel mutation D1790G linked to the long-QT syndrome. Circulation 2000; 102: 921–5.
36. Priori SG, Napolitano C, Schwartz PJ et al. The elusive link between LQT3 and Brugada syndrome: the role of flecainide challenge. Circulation 2000; 102: 945–7.
37. Brugada P, Brugada J. Right bundle branch block, persistent ST segment elevation and sudden cardiac death: a distinct clinical and electrocardiographic syndrome. A multicenter report. J Am Coll Cardiol 1992; 20: 1391–6.
38. Priori SG. Foretelling the future in Brugada syndrome: do we have the crystal ball? J Cardiovasc Electrophysiol 2001; 12: 1008–9.
39. Priori SG, Grillo M, Napolitano C et al. Epidemiology of Brugada syndrome: a prospective evaluation of 192 individuals. Circulation 104(suppl II), 540. 2001. Ref Type: Abstract.
40. Priori SG, Napolitano C. Should patients with an asymptomatic Brugada electrocardiogram undergo pharmacological and electrophysiological testing? Circulation 2005; 112: 279–92.

41. Brugada J, Brugada R, Brugada P. Right bundle-branch block and ST-segment elevation in leads V1 through V3: a marker for sudden death in patients without demonstrable structural heart disease. Circulation 1998; 97: 457–60.
42. Brugada J, Brugada R, Antzelevitch C et al. Long-term follow-up of individuals with the electrocardiographic pattern of right bundle-branch block and ST-segment elevation in precordial leads V1 to V3. Circulation 2002; 105: 73–8.
43. Antzelevitch C, Brugada P, Borggrefe M et al. Brugada syndrome. Report of the Second Consensus Conference. Endorsed by the Heart Rhythm Society and the European Heart Rhythm Association. Circulation 2005; 111: 659–70.
44. Chen Q, Kirsch GE, Zhang D et al. Genetic basis and molecular mechanism for idiopathic ventricular fibrillation. Nature 1998; 392: 293–6.
45. Priori SG, Napolitano C, Gasparini M et al. Natural history of Brugada syndrome. insights for risk stratification and management. Circulation 2002; 105: 1342–7.
46. Valdivia CR, Ackerman MJ, Tester DJ et al. A novel SCN5A arrhythmia mutation, M1766L, with expression defect rescued by mexiletine. Cardiovasc Res 2002; 55: 279–89.
47. Brugada P, Brugada R, Mont L et al. Natural history of Brugada syndrome: the prognostic value of programmed electrical stimulation of the heart. J Cardiovasc Electrophysiol 2003; 14: 455–7.
48. Atarashi H, Ogawa S, Harumi K et al. Three-year follow-up of patients with right bundle branch block and ST segment elevation in the right precordial leads: Japanese Registry of Brugada Syndrome. Idiopathic Ventricular Fibrillation Investigators. J Am Coll Cardiol 2001; 37: 1916–20.
49. Eckardt L, Probst V, Smits JPP et al. Long-term prognosis of individuals with right precordial ST-segment-elevation Brugada syndrome. Circulation 2005; 111: 257–63.
50. Antzelevitch C. The Brugada syndrome: ionic basis and arrhythmia mechanisms. J Cardiovasc Electrophysiol 2001; 12: 268–72.
51. Yan GX, Antzelevitch C. Cellular basis for the Brugada syndrome and other mechanisms of arrhythmogenesis associated with ST-segment elevation. Circulation 1999; 100: 1660–6.
52. Belhassen B, Viskin S, Fish R et al. Effects of electrophysiologic-guided therapy with class IA antiarrhythmic drugs on the long-term outcome of patients with idiopathic ventricular fibrillation with or without the Brugada syndrome. J Cardiovasc Electrophysiol 1999; 10: 1301–12.
53. Hermida JS, Denjoy I, Clerc J et al. Hydroquinidine therapy in Brugada syndrome. J Am Coll Cardiol 2004; 43: 1853–60.
54. Belhassen B, Glick A, Viskin S. Efficacy of quinidine in high-risk patients with Brugada syndrome. Circulation 2004; 110: 1731–7.
55. Freestone B, Lip GY. Tedisamil: a new novel antiarrhythmic. Expert Opin Investig Drugs 2004; 13: 151–60.
56. Tsuchiya T, Ashikaga K, Honda T, Arita M. Prevention of ventricular fibrillation by cilostazol, an oral phosphodiesterase inhibitor, in a patient with Brugada syndrome. J Cardiovasc Electrophysiol 2002; 13: 698–701.
57. Valdivia CR, Tester DJ, Rok BA et al. A trafficking defective, Brugada syndrome-causing SCN5A mutation rescued by drugs. Cardiovasc Res 2004; 62: 53–62.
58. Baroudi G, Pouliot V, Denjoy I et al. Novel mechanism for Brugada syndrome: defective surface localization of an SCN5A mutant (R1432G). Circ Res 2001; 88: E78–E83.
59. Coumel P, Fidelle J, Lucet V, Attuel P, Bouvrain Y. Catecholaminergic-induced severe ventricular arrhythmias with Adams–Stokes syndrome in children: report of four cases. Br Heart J 1978; 40: 28–37.
60. Swan H, Piippo K, Viitasalo M et al. Arrhythmic disorder mapped to chromosome 1q42-q43 causes malignant polymorphic ventricular tachycardia in structurally normal hearts. J Am Coll Cardiol 1999; 34: 2035–42.
61. Priori SG, Napolitano C, Memmi M et al. Clinical and molecular characterization of patients with catecholaminergic polymorphic ventricular tachycardia. Circulation 2002; 106: 69–74.

62. Cerrone M, Colombi B, Bloise R et al. Clinical and molecular characterization of a large cohort of patients affected with catecholaminergic polymorphic ventricular tachycardia. Circulation 110[17], 552(supplII)(Abstr.). 2004. Ref Type: Abstract.
63. Leenhardt A, Lucet V, Denjoy I et al. Catecholaminergic polymorphic ventricular tachycardia in children. A 7-year follow-up of 21 patients. Circulation 1995; 91: 1512–9.
64. Priori SG, Napolitano C, Tiso N et al. Mutations in the cardiac ryanodine receptor gene (hRyR2) underlie catecholaminergic polymorphic ventricular tachycardia. Circulation 2001; 103: 196–200.
65. Jiang D, Xiao B, Zhang L, Chen SR. Enhanced basal activity of a cardiac $Ca^{2+}$ release channel (ryanodine receptor) mutant associated with ventricular tachycardia and sudden death. Circ Res 2002; 91: 218–25.
66. Wehrens XH, Lehnart SE, Huang F et al. FKBP12.6 deficiency and defective calcium release channel (ryanodine receptor) function linked to exercise-induced sudden cardiac death. Cell 2003; 113: 829–40.
67. Lahat H, Eldar M, Levy-Nissenbaum E et al. Autosomal recessive catecholamine- or exercise-induced polymorphic ventricular tachycardia. Circulation 2001; 103: 2822–7.
68. Postma AV, Denjoy I, Hoorntje TM et al. Absence of calsequestrin 2 causes severe forms of catecholaminergic polymorphic ventricular tachycardia. Circ Res 2002; 91: e21–e6.
69. Napolitano C, Priori SG. Catecholaminergic polymorphic ventricular tachycardia. In: Zipes DP, Jalife J, eds. Cardiac Electrophysiology. 4th edn. Philadelphia: Elsevier, 2004: 633–9.
70. Lehnart SE, Wehrens XHT, Laitinen PJ et al. Sudden death in familial polymorphic ventricular tachycardia associated with calcium release channel (ryanodine receptor) leak. Circulation 2004; 109: 3208–14.
71. Yano M, Kobayashi S, Kohno M et al. FKBP12.6-mediated stabilization of calcium-release channel (ryanodine receptor) as a novel therapeutic strategy against heart failure. Circulation 2003; 107: 477–84.
72. Wehrens XH, Lehnart SE, Reiken SR et al. Protection from cardiac arrhythmia through ryanodine receptor-stabilizing protein calstabin2. Science 2004; 304: 292–6.
73. Cerrone M, Colombi B, Santoro M et al. Bidirectional ventricular tachycardia and fibrillation elicited in a knock-in mouse model carrier of a mutation in the cardiac ryanodine receptor (RyR2). Circ Res 2005; 96: e77–e82.
74. Johns DC, Nuss HB, Chiamvimonvat N et al. Adenovirus-mediated expression of a voltage-gated potassium channel in vitro (rat cardiac myocytes) and in vivo (rat liver). A novel strategy for modifying excitability. J Clin Invest 1995; 96: 1152–8.
75. Nuss HB, Johns DC, Kaab S et al. Reversal of potassium channel deficiency in cells from failing hearts by adenoviral gene transfer: a prototype for gene therapy for disorders of cardiac excitability and contractility. Gene Ther 1996; 3: 900–12.
76. Donahue JK, Kikuchi K, Sasano T. Gene therapy for cardiac arrhythmias. Trends Cardiovasc Med 2005; 15: 219–24.
77. Ennis IL, Li RA, Murphy AM, Marban E, Nuss HB. Dual gene therapy with SERCA1 and Kir2.1 abbreviates excitation without suppressing contractility. J Clin Invest 2002; 109: 393–400.
78. Donahue JK, Heldman AW, Fraser H et al. Focal modification of electrical conduction in the heart by viral gene transfer. Nat Med 2000; 6: 1395–8.
79. Bauer A, McDonald AD, Nasir K et al. Inhibitory G protein overexpression provides physiologically relevant heart rate control in persistent atrial fibrillation. Circulation 2004; 110: 3115–20.
80. Murata M, Cingolani E, McDonald AD, Donahue JK, Marban E. Creation of a genetic calcium channel blocker by targeted gem gene transfer in the heart. Circ Res 2004; 95: 398–405.
81. Potapova I, Plotnikov AN, Danilo P Jr et al. Human mesenchymal stem cells as a gene delivery system to create cardiac pacemakers. Circulation 2004; 94: 952–9.

# Index

Page numbers in *italics* refer to tables and figures.